DEMENTIA BLUES

To Crawb, the truest of friends, Love, Stu

BY STU JENKS

FEZZIWIG PRESS 2011

Dementia Blues

First Edition

ISBN: 978-0-9842891-4-1

Printed in Iowa, USA

Fezziwig Press
PO Box 161
Tucson, Arizona 85702

www.stujenks.com

Fezziwig Press logo design by Julie Unruh.

TABLE OF CONTENTS

Dedicated to Annie Gordon

WHAT YOU HAVE IS WHAT HE FOUND

Introduction by Bo Petersen

Well, how it happened was I wanted to go to Florida for the weekend. My brother was in school there, lived out on the Indian River and had a beer ball game planned. (You don't want to know.) My last class was Thursday morning, and my first class the next week would be Monday at noon. It had taken me until junior year, second semester, to rig this kind of user-friendly class load and I meant to use it.

There were two issues.

This was the 1970's. Thumbing was a way of life if you were in school and didn't have a car. But the Indian River was 630 miles down I-95, the bad ass pro road of the East. I didn't hesitate to stick out my thumb on most North Carolina roads, but I-95 was a different animal. I wanted a second. Only a few people I knew would do it. The all-over-the-place found object artiste of Chapel Hill was the first one. Naturally.

The second issue was a little more ticklish. Getting to I-95 from Chapel Hill meant going through Smithfield, and in those days the road to Smithfield had one of those huge, eyesnatching KKK Wants You billboards. Neither Stu or I was real big on strolling underneath it with our thumbs out.

Mary Jenks took care of that one. Stu's mom drove us to the interstate ramp.

Mary Jenks always was a handful, not shy about laying into Stu or anybody else over whatever irked her at the moment. But she didn't lecture us. She pressed enough to realize we had at least a clue what we were doing and that we were going to do it with or without her OK. She took us to the interstate and told us she would come get us when we got back. You had to love the optimism.

We grabbed our backpacks, walked on down through a stand of pines and stuck out our thumbs. Just like that, we got picked up by a trucker on a Quebec to Miami run who was bored enough of the twice-a-week haul to put up with us.

We ended up Sunday on I-95 outside of Melbourne, Fla., trying to thumb home and watching car after car zoom by with drivers and passengers giving us the sort of terrified glance you would give a guy standing there with a chainsaw. We had no idea that a serial killer down in Miami was operating as a hitchhiker and police had just alerted motorists to Be On the Look Out. All we got was sun poisoning and—in one of those double entendres that you could twist into a harbinger of either of our careers—a warning ticket for "walking on the expressway."

Anyhow, it was Mary Jenks who picked us up Monday morning at the Raleigh airport, drove us back to school and dropped me off outside Greenlaw Hall just in time to stroll into class.

Mary has always been conflicted, so she tends to leave others with conflicted feelings about her. She is much more like Stu than he might be ready to acknowledge, and it's tormenting in this book to see the glimpses of her coming through the dementia. What it does to him is right there bleeding on the page.

Stu has always been off somewhere. He lit out from school one time to hike the Nolichucky Gorge in the Appalachians in the dead of winter, with no real gear for the weather. He planned to sleep in his beater Karmann Ghia, which by this time had a rust hole under the passenger seat big enough that you could watch the road zing past. He gave me a lift to Hickory, where my family lived, and I sat hunched shivering in the warmest coat I had, with my feet up on the seat to keep them out of the cold blast. That one, I think, ended when he was forced to turn around on an iced-over mountain road. The Ghia wasn't your ideal all-terrain vehicle.

Stu has made a name as a "mythic" photographer. To my mind his strength is earthier, rooted in landscapes and people who fascinate him.

I like to tell the True Fact that I lived with 11 different people in college after first semester freshman year. Every one of them dropped out of school; every one of them dropped out of school while they were living with me. Hell, one of them did twice. The found object artiste was among them, and maybe was the one you would have picked to go if you knew us back then. And, yeah, go he did, off in a lot of different directions.

What you have is what he found.

Bo Petersen
Reporter, *The Post and Courier*, Charleston, South Carolina
January, 2011

[Note from Stu: I didn't drop out of college. I flunked out while living with Bo Petersen. But I went back during the summer sessions, got my grades up and graduated from the University of North Carolina at Chapel Hill in 1979 with a BFA in Studio Art.

And if you ask me nice, I'll tell you about what happened at Indian River that weekend with Bo, but I won't write about it here, even though I'm pretty sure the statutes of limitations have expired by now.]

TWO THINGS TO TELL YOU

RICHMOND, VIRGINIA • SPR NG, 2001

Mary just left the hospital room to talk with a nurse, her eyes still puffy from crying.

Stuart sits in a chair, next to his bed, reading the paper.

I'm thinking about going outside to have a smoke.

It's raining in Richmond.

The news is bad.

A few hours ago, Dad was sent into a small operating room to have a procedure done on his chest, but when the surgeon read the new x-rays, he found that the cancer had spread and he didn't even bother to open Dad up. Both lungs, around his heart, beginning to go down his left arm. A lot of cancer, everywhere. The doctor simply stitched up the small incision and came out to see Mom and I in the waiting area. As soon as he entered the room, I knew.

"Mrs. Jenks, performing the procedure on Stuart will only make him uncomfortable. We didn't do the procedure. I'm sorry. There is nothing more we can do. Just make Stuart as comfortable as you can," said the doctor.

"Oh God," said Mom, beginning to cry.

"How long does he have, Doc?" I said.

"I can't really say," The surgeon said nervously.

"Ballpark, Doc. I'm not going to hold you to it," I asked.

"Could be three months. Could be a year," he said.

I sensed three months was closer to the truth.

"What can we do?" Mom said through her tears.

"Just make him comfortable. And you all can go home tomorrow. I'm sorry, Mrs. Jenks," he said. The doctor truly looked very sad that he couldn't do more for Stuart, for Mary, for me.

"Thanks Doc for all that you did," I said.

The surgeon rose and left, and Mom and I just sat in the overstuffed chairs, not saying much.

"Mom, are you all right? I'm going out for a smoke. You be OK for a few minutes?" I said.

"I'm OK, son. Go ahead."

"I'll be right back."

I go down a flight of stairs, exit the hospital and stand out front. I light a Camel Filter. It's misting, just beginning to rain. I begin to cry. I look around to see if anyone's walking up to the entrance. No one. I then allow myself to cry a little harder.

"Well, that's it." I whisper to myself.

"That's it."

Up in the hospital room, Dad and I are alone. Mary is still out in the hall doing something. Stuart has been given the bad news that the cancer has spread and there is nothing more to be done. He and I talk about heading home to The River. No talk about dying in a few months. Just small talk between father and son.

Then Dad surprises me.

"Stu, I need to talk with you."

All the blood drains from my face. What in God's name does Dad need to talk with me about? He usually avoids all heavy discussions, but then again, he is dying now. Is he going to ask how I plan to take care of Mom? Does he have some words of wisdom for me to live by? (That would be a first.) Is he angry at me for something? What?

"You want to talk now?" I say.

"Just a little later," Stuart says, "I'll let your mother know that I want to talk with you."

"OK."

Mary comes back and Dad mentions that he wants to talk with me alone for just a few minutes. Mom looks a little nervous. She hates being left out.

"All right," says Mom, "I'll go down to the cafeteria and get a little something to eat"

"We won't be long, Mary," Stuart says.

Mom leaves.

"I just have two things to tell you," Dad says.

I'm hardly breathing.

"One, you know the Huckster Wagon? Well, your mother tells me you want to have it."

"Yeah, I do," I say.

[The Huckster Wagon is the Model A Ford Pickup Truck my father rebuilt with love and care a number of years ago. A beautiful tan four cylinder vehicle. I imagine myself driving it on dusty desert roads in Arizona. Dad put it up on blocks in Raleigh ten years ago before he moved up to Virginia to retire.]

"I'll be happy to sign over the title to you, son. That's no problem, but don't hang on to it on my account. It may be more trouble to you then it's worth. You've got to get it out to Arizona first and then you'll have to have it garaged. It's sort of like that old joke about the two happiest days when you own a boat. The day you buy it and the day you sell it."

I laugh.

"Don't worry," I tell Dad, "I won't keep it just because of you, but I would like to have it."

"All right," he says. "Before you leave to go back to Tucson, we'll go up to the Post Office in Farnham, and have the title signed over to you and notarized. How's that sound?"

"Sounds good to me"

"Second thing," Dad continues, "is don't take any shit from your sister!"

I laugh even louder this time.

"You know, Pamela is such a selfish....well, anyway....just don't take any shit from her."

Smiling I say, "Thanks Dad. No, no....I won't take any shit from her."

"Good," he says.

That was it. No profound revelation from God that he received in a dream. No words of reprimand for things done or undone. No apologies for any past actions. Just don't keep the Huckster simply in memory of your father, and don't take any crap from Pamela.

Then again, those are pretty powerful words of wisdom. I only wish he'd given me the green light on Pamela about 40 years ago.

Going home to Tucson tomorrow. We're all back at The River House now. We're exhausted. I go upstairs to my bedroom to start packing for my flight in the morning, when I spy my mother and father sleeping together in the other guest room. I tiptoe to get my 35 mm Pentax, come back to the door and take their picture as they sleep. Mom snuggles up to Dad. Dad on his back, his foot on the bed rail. Both fully clothed with their shoes still on. Mary and Stuart look so sweet, like newlyweds, but with an ease of having slept with each other for over 50 years.

I look closely at Dad. He looks old now, after all the many procedures, all the years of chemo, all the cancer. He is dying. I can see it.

I quietly turn, go back to my guest room, and put the camera away.

I sigh and wipe a tear away.

I've always been someone who cries easily, but now, I seem to cry all the time.

Then again, I have a reason to cry.

THE PINE FOREST SPIRAL

MOTHERSHEAD NECK, VIRGINIA • SUMMER, 2001

I received the call late Saturday night.

"Stu, It's time. You need to come now," said Mom.

On Monday, I told work I needed to go.

On Tuesday, I was on a plane.

On Tuesday night, I drove up Route 3 in a white rental pickup truck, took a right on State Road 608, drove through Mothershead Neck, and up the drive to The River House. My sister's car was already there. All the lights were on in the house. It was just after ten o'clock.

I walked into the house and went straight to my Dad's room.

"Well, Stuart, look who's here!" Mom says.

My dad's lying flat in bed, his eyes closed.

I grab my father's hand.

"Hey Dad, how are you doing?"

Dad opens his eyes.

"Well, hey there son. Glad…well…glad you're here."

"Me too, Dad. You hangin' in?"

"Yep. How was your flight?"

"It was OK."

He's noticeably smaller in the legs and arms then he was three months ago. His left arm's very swollen though, and above his left pectoral muscle grows a large white bandage that covers a cancerous growth as big as your fist.

"Well, I'm going to get my bags out of the truck," I say.

"Oh…Ok". He squeezes my hand again and I squeeze back. I look up from Dad to look at my sister and mother. They look wiped out. I turn and go outside to get my bags.

It's the first week in August, 2001.

I'm home to help my father die.

Hospice consists of my mother Mary, my sister Pamela, and I. That's it. A nurse comes to the house every other day to change Stuart's chest bandage, but she leaves soon after. Mom says Dad doesn't want hospice, but I think she's the one who doesn't want strangers in the house. So it's just the three of us. Three people who don't really get along that well, but who love Stuart enough to be here to help.

Pamela and I trade shifts on who will get up in the middle of the night and lift Dad when he needs lifting, or to change his leaky diapers when they need changing, or to simply help Mom in some other way. On nights when it is my turn, I wake quickly after Mary yells for me to come downstairs. Every time she yells 'Stu!' from the bottom of the stairs, I listen to the tone in her voice to see if it is an emergency or not. Mostly it's just to lift Dad's frail body or to help clean him up.

During the day, there's more lifting Dad up. A lot of scooting him up in the bed. A lot of pillow-fluffing. A lot of feeding him fresh cantaloupe by hand. A lot of helping him drink Gatorade with a straw. A lot of us just sitting with him while he sleeps. None of us sleep well except Dad.

A week passes.

There have only been a few times in my life when I knew I was in the right place, doing the right thing, with the right people, at the right time. Being here, now, with Dad, is one of those times.

A baby monitor, its On/Off light glowing red, sits on a bedside table near my Dad. The other monitor is in the living room. When I go outside to the pier for a break, I take a walkie-talkie with me if I'm suddenly needed. Usually I get buzzed at the pier to come help lift Dad, but there's another call I hope I never get.

See, Dad's pectoral muscle cancer has spread to his lungs and now has also surrounded his heart and his coronary arteries. There's a possibility, we've been told by the nurse, that Dad may die by having one of his coronary arteries rupture.

That he might bleed out.

If that happens, blood will fly out of his mouth and nose under high pressure, spraying the room, the walls, the bed, and he will be dead within seconds. We've placed bath towels all around the bedroom to put over his mouth and face if he starts to bleed out. This is our worst fear. We pray he dies in his sleep.

Every time the walkie-talkie gets keyed and I hear my mother's voice, I wonder if she's calling to tell me that there's blood everywhere.

This morning, I've walked to the little pine forest next to the house. My father planted this forest fifteen years ago. They were little seedlings less than a foot high back then. Now they are twenty-foot-tall pines, all equal distance apart, all in neat rows. Just like my Dad to be so precise in his planting. A thick bed of needles covers the forest floor. I slowly stroll through his forest. A beautiful place, a wonderful gift my father has given to the Earth. He didn't have those kind of noble thoughts when he planted the trees, but they're true just the same.

I see a space in between some of the trees. I reach down and touch the pine needles. I have an idea.

Bending over, I begin to form a ridge from the pine needles with my hands. I slowly walk backwards as I fluff the needles, making a spiral on the forest floor. It takes a little time to get it right, to get it precise. I am my father's son.

After I'm done, I walk into the spiral and then walk out again. Spiral in, spiral out. The journey upward, the journey down. A little gift for my Dad. I'll photograph it in a few days, but not right now.

I pray to God to give my Dad an easy death. A death without exploding arteries and gushing blood. A death with some peace and little pain. A death that won't hurt him or traumatize his family very much.

"Please, God, if you could do this, I would be so grateful." I don't expect God to intervene but it would be nice if the worst didn't happen.

I then walk into an old shed not far away, in search of an offering for the spiral. I find it right away. I walk outside to Father's Forest and place my prayer offering in the very center of the spiral.

A 40-year-old solid wood croquet ball with a red stripe painted around its center.

STU & STUART SLEEPING

MOTHERSHEAD NECK, VIRGINIA • FALL, 2001

Dad's making the death rattle now. We've turned off the baby monitor for Dad's moans and groans drive my sister and mother crazy. But not me. He's just fighting to die and I'm silently cheering him on. And I don't mind sitting with him.

I place my pinhole camera on top of the TV. I open the shutter and return to the comfy chair beside his bed. He's not so noisy this afternoon. I have never been so tired in all my life. But I'm happy in a way, living an archetype and all that. That sounds so cold. I don't mean it to be. Just saying that millions, if not billions of humans over the past 50,000 years have sat beside a dying parent and been with them as they went to the Other Side. I'm one of those people now. Happy to be here. Don't forget to tip the waitresses.

It's late afternoon. I'm slaphappy. Think I'll catch a couple winks. I'm sure Mom will wake me soon enough for something. Better get some sleep while I can.

I stare at the camera on the TV and then look over at Dad. He should show up on the negative but me? Don't know.

And at 'Don't know,' I'm sound asleep.

[Dad died early Labor Day morning, September 4th, 2001, a few days after I took that pinhole photograph. He didn't bleed out. He was in very little pain. He died in his sleep with his wife by his side and his two children, happily chatting on the front porch. He was 79 years old.]

OUR CONFEDERATE DEAD

TUCSON, ARIZONA • WINTER SOLSTICE, 2007

5:30 a.m. Might as well do laundry. I'm not going to be able to get back to sleep for I had the oddest dream.

I dreamt I was dead.

Somebody once told me that you can't die in a dream. They were wrong.

I was my age now. I died. I remember going from living to dead. Don't know what I died of, but I felt it. Traveling from living to dead.

I still had some things to say and do, even though I was dead. I was keeping a list. I was reading the list. I was walking around Tucson with a woman. She reminded me of someone I knew. She was tall, blond, attractive, in her 40's or 50's. She didn't talk much but was with me the whole time.

I felt pretty good just after I had died, but as time went on, in the dream, I felt worse and worse. After a while, I couldn't talk anymore. I had no energy. I felt like I was slightly choking. I was really sad I couldn't communicate with my friends anymore, with this beautiful woman anymore.

Then I didn't want to be dead any longer. But I was dead. The woman I had been walking with said she was sorry. I couldn't speak.

I was so upset. I didn't want to be dead. I wanted to be alive again. I want to be alive.

Then I woke up.

I get up from my bed, stunned but oddly happy. Disoriented, hardly able to walk but strangely buzzing. I took a bath. (Odd, for I never take baths in the morning.) I pack up my dirty clothes and head for the apartment complex's laundry room. Still dark and chilly. Air hits me hard in the face and it is wonderful. I think of the living, changing, aging body of Stu: more weight around the middle, less hair on top, a wrinkled face. My vanity would have cared yesterday. But not now. I'm just so happy to be alive, to not be walking around Tucson in a dead, silent, painful body.

I pray I always remember this dream, but I know I won't.

COMMON

HARRIMAN, TENNESSEE • SPRING, 2008

Thought driving Miss Daisy across the country would be fun. Really thought Mary would enjoy the trip, spending time with Annie and I, staying in nice hotels, seeing the USA in our Chevrolet. Boy, was I wrong.

Mom called Annie common today. A peasant. Someone without intuition. I don't think I've ever seen Annie so mad. And Mary wants to go back to Virginia now. I told her she can't. She's coming to Arizona to live near me. Odd she would want to go back to the Northern Neck, after she begged me for two years to let her move to Arizona.

When Mom doesn't get her way, you are wrong. Mary is never wrong. I've never heard Mom say she's sorry. Not even once in my life. I'm not exaggerating. If you disagree with Mary, you hate her. If you are angry at some behavior of hers, you hate her. If you ask for something she doesn't want to give, you hate her. This is nothing new. But what is new is the intensity of Mom's protests. She seems out of her mind. It's like she's in a nightmare of her own making, but it's all my fault. Then again, she's always been hysterical, even when she's having a good time. But this is more. A lot more. And I don't think she's really seen anything from the highway. No Red Buds in bloom. No Blue Ridge Mountain vistas. She just talks and complains and complains some more, as she stares blankly out the window. It's gotten so bad that Annie and I take Mary on alternate days. Monday: With Annie in the Buick. Tuesday: With me in the Penske Truck. Wednesday: Back to Annie. We just can't handle Mary for more than one day at a time. It's sad. We just put Mary to bed a little while ago. Annie's calmed down a little. So have I. It's been one weird day. I saw this wild billboard when we parked the car and truck this afternoon. Now it's night and the sign's brightly lit. Reminds me of an image by Blake Hines. Think I'll shoot it and put my own spin on it. Take it a step in a different direction. And photographing gives me something to do, rather than worry about what lies ahead for my mother and I.

MARY AT THE CADILLAC RANCH

AMARILLO, TEXAS • SPRING, 2008

Prairie wind's blowing like a son of a gun. The Buick and Penske are parked over there. Annie walks with Mary toward the Cadillacs. Leaves Mom by herself, while she walks around. I take a picture of Mary alone with the sculpture. Nice shot. She looks confused.

"Mom?" I yell over the wind.

She turns her head. I take another shot. Mary doesn't say anything. She's hardly talking at all today, Annie says. Not like the other night in Arkansas.

We're all checked in at the Holiday Inn in who-knows-where Arkansas. Off we go, in the Buick, to get some dinner somewhere. Mary's in the back. Annie's next to me. I'm driving.

"Where are we going to eat?" asks Mary.

"Well, I don't know. Maybe that Chinese place over..."

"Why are we here? I want to go back to Virginia! I really need to eat something now! Are you listening to me? I just don't know!" says Mary.

"Mom, please don't interrupt."

"I never interrupt!" yells Mom.

"Yes you do, Mary," says Annie. "You interrupt all the time."

Yikes. Annie's not usually so demonstrative. Usually keeps her opinions to herself.

"I do not! I do not!" Mary yells, "I hate it here! I can't stand it here! I can't! You're not listening to me!"

"Oh, Mom, I..."

"You never listen to me! I need to eat! Where are we going? I can't stand this! I can't!" she yells.

She doesn't stop talking. Just goes on and on. Yelling and talking and yelling some more. She's pitching a fit and I'm not even sure why. Finally, I put my foot down like you would with a petulant child.

"Mom, you need to calm down. I'm not taking you anywhere unless you calm down. We're not going into any restaurant with you like this."

Mary starts to cry. Yelling through the tears.

I've had enough.

"Mom, I'm going back to the hotel. We'll get something to eat in the room."

"I'll die if I go back there!" she screams.

"No you won't. But I can't take you out like this."

"I'll die! I'll die!"

I turn the car around and head back to the hotel.

"I need to get out of here!" Mary yells. She reaches for her door handle. Holy shit!

I push the Master Door Lock Button, but instead of locking all the doors, I unlock them all. Mom opens the back door and tries to jump out of the moving car. I put on the brakes and pull over into a parking lot. Annie leaps out of the car and runs back to Mary's door. She slams it.

"Mary! You get back in that car right now!" Annie screams. I didn't know Annie could yell that loud. Hmm. Oddly, I'm feeling quite calm in the center of this storm.

Mary continues to cry as we return to the hotel. At the hotel, she first refuses to get out of the car then relents. We take her upstairs, put her to bed and tell Mom we need some time by ourselves. I look at Mary's face. She knows she's screwed up. Annie and I then hit a Waffle House, eats some eggs, and call my sister Pamela to report what we soon coin 'The Arkansas Incident.' Pamela's not surprised. But we sure are. Mary can be a royal pain in the neck, but she's never tried to jump out of a moving vehicle before.

The next morning, Mary walks up to Annie, before climbing into the truck with me. I have Mom today.

"Annie," Mom says, "I just want you to know that I would have never jumped out of the car. I just needed some air."

"You scared the crap out of me, Mary," Annie says.

Mom looks down at the ground. She doesn't say she's sorry, but she does look a little embarrassed.

"OK, Mom. Let me help you in the truck. You're with me today," I say as cheerfully as I can. And off we go.

I take one last exposure of my mother with the Cadillacs. She looks cold. It is a bit nippy here in Amarillo, with the wind and all.

"You want to go back to the car, Mom?" I ask.

"Yes."

"I'll take her," Annie says, leading Mary back to the Buick. She has Mom today.

"Thanks," I say. "I won't be long."

Just want to take it all in. The cars, the wind, everything.

I turn and look toward my Mother. She looks so pitiful. I slowly shake my head.

SHOOT YOU MYSELF

TUCSON, ARIZONA • SPRING, 2009

Mary sits on a plush leather sofa at House Number Three at Crossroads Adult Care Center, in Tucson, Arizona. This is where she lives. She's not having a good day.

Mom sold The River House and Father's Forest in 2003 so she could invest the money and simply live. (My father didn't believe in life insurance. That's kind of fucked up, if you ask me. You'd think he would want to leave his wife of 50-plus years some cash, but he didn't.) We moved Mary out to the desert a year ago, much to my initial protests, but I now know it was the right thing to do, for we soon discovered that Mary had a very fast-progressing dementia. Within six months of her arrival in Tucson, she went from Independent Living to Assisted Living to Nursing Care to Kino Psych Ward to Crossroads Adult Care.

Today, she's fully aware of her predicament. She knows she will never get better. She wants to die. I don't blame her.

"You know, Son," she says, "I've made peace with Death."

"I know, Mom," I say. You can tell she has.

"I'm ready to go," she says.

I hate that she suffers. I hate the mystery of it all. I doubt she'll die this year. Probably next. Jesus.

"Mom," I say matter-of-factly, "If I thought I could get away with it, I'd take you out in the desert and shoot you myself."

She reaches over and pats my arm.

"That's so sweet of you,' she says, "but you'll get caught."

I laugh out loud.

"Yeah, Mom. You're probably right."

"But it was sweet of you to offer."

"You're welcome, Mom."

BRISTLECONE HOOP DANCE

THE WHITE MOUNTAINS, CALIFORNIA
SUMMER, 2009

Spin a line of blue LED Christmas lights. Make a circle. Hear the whoosh of the wire traveling through the air. While the wire of lights spin, click on the light's switch with my thumb. Spin the lit lights about seven revolutions. Switch the lights off while still making the circle. Come to rest. Take two steps sideways. Settle. Spin the line again. Make the circle again. Repeat the process. Take two more side steps uphill. Do this at least fifteen times until I'm sure I'm out of the frame.

The Rollei's with me but I'm not using it. Lately, the Canon 5D Mark II has been my camera of choice. It's working very well tonight.

I'm barely here, mostly in my head, in another city, with a woman. I force myself back into the forest. Trying the Spiritual Trick-Fuck. It's not working.

I check the back of the Canon to see if I got the shot. Almost. Need to spin just a bit higher off the ground. I go back to the ancient Bristlecone and do my side-stepping dance one more time.

Focusing on making this image takes my mind off my broken heart. It's been a rough couple of days. Frankly, it's been hell.

We haven't been lovers in over a year and a half, and even then, it wasn't right. She wanted a long-term partner, and I wasn't into that at the time. I smoked and she has family who has died of cancer. I'm intense, she's pretty quiet. Sadly, now, I'm more open to living the rest of my days with someone, with her. I'm seriously thinking of becoming smoke free, and I now understand the blessing of keeping my mouth shut sometimes. But it's too late. She has moved on. She has moved far away. We are still close friends, but I recently found out that she is dating someone. It may get serious, she said. I was cool on the phone, more than open to staying friends with her and I told her so, but then minutes later, after I hung up, I felt something I haven't felt in decades. I'm jealous. Insanely jealous. I'm the jealous ex-lover. Fuck me.

I've been talking to God almost constantly as I drive today. God, help me to let go of her. God, help me to not think about all of this, all the time. God, help me to be a good man. God, help me.

Just south of Bishop, I ask God the big question, the simplest question, the truest question:

"God, what is all of this really about?"

The quiet still voice said only seven words. I began to cry. I had to pull over I was quaking so hard. I haven't cried like that since my last Breathwork experience.

"You just want her to come home," said the voice.

Through my tears, I get out: "That's true. I just want her to come home. I just want you to come home."

I finish my spinning, my hoop dancing. Judging from what I can see on the back of the 5D, I think I have the shot, but I won't really know for sure until I download the digital negative onto my Apple at home. There is still some mystery in digital photography

I pack up my gear but I don't leave the Bristlecone Pine Forest right away. I walk around the Ancients for a while. I visit an old tree I met last year, a 3,000-year-old man just down that hill. It was good to hug him again. I sit on an outcropping of rock near the tree I just photographed and drink some water. It's three miles back to the car, and all of my grieving from the last few days has tuckered me out. My gear's heavy but it's my heart that's weighting me down. I drink some more water, drop my head in exhaustion and cry some more.

She's not coming home, Stu. She's not coming home.

TEARFUL MARY

TUCSON, ARIZONA • SUMMER, 2009

"What I don't like about it is..." Mary says, her voice trailing off.

She sees something outside of her window. A car? A bird? It doesn't matter. It's enough for her to lose her train of thought.

"What I need you to know is..." she says a minute later.

"I can't seem to find..." Mom says after a while.

"I'm not unhappy but I don't know where I am," she says, her first completed sentence since I arrived today.

She looks very unhappy. She is unhappy, and angry and sad too.

Mom's good days are when the dementia is strongest. She knows me. She's happy to be in bed. She's happy with how well the staff treats her. She loves the house. She listens and responds to what I've said, with love and kindness. She thinks she will die soon, and is at peace with that.

Mom's bad days are when the dementia weakens. She knows that she can't walk, can't go to bathroom by herself, can't leave the house, can barely feed herself. She's knows her mind is going. She aware she can't finish sentences and it makes her mad. She knows there is nothing she can do to make things better, and that makes her sad. She tries to listen to me but gets lost in her own hopelessness. I don't blame her at all for that. She thinks she's going to live for a very long time. She's afraid of that Very Long Time. She cries sometimes.

Mary's having a bad day today.

As I walk to my car after our visit, I shake my head.

"Jesus, God. Please take this woman," I whisper to the wind.

I WANT MY MOMMA

TUCSON, ARIZONA • FALL, 2009

Mary sees things that are not there. Dad. Other men. Boys from her high school in Alexandria, Virginia. Her mother, Nannie. Her grandfather, Daddy Saum.

Mostly these visions don't scare her. She just looks at them with wonder. Frankly, I don't know all she sees because I only ask her when I'm there, and when I think it's a good time to ask. I'm sure she sees a lot more people and things than any of us will ever know.

Mary's condition has worsened. For a few days, she had a very hard time eating anything. Now, she can eat a little. For a few days, she slept all the time. Now, she sleeps about 20 hours a day. Just a couple weeks ago, she could follow a conservation, and respond with kindness and attention. Now, at best, she just goes away as I talk to some place where I cannot follow.

I walk into her room, this morning. She's asleep. Jessica told me earlier that Mom has eaten some pudding. I said, "Good," but I didn't really mean it. (If she completely stops eating, she will be dead within a month. Her suffering will end.) I grab an old wooden chair we brought from Virginia, and place it beside her bed. I raise her bed with the electric controls, so I can easily talk with her. She doesn't really wake up. Her eyes open, but she doesn't really see. I say, "Hello, Mom," but she doesn't really hear. Then she begins to say one phrase over and over, very softly, in her strong Virginia accent. Most people wouldn't understand her. I know exactly what she's saying.

"I want my Momma. I want my Momma, I want my Momma...."

I touch her hand. I start to cry. I cry hard. Her bedroom door's closed to the rest of the house, so I let fly. I cry for her, for me, for everything. I don't know where some things end and others begin anymore. My deep grief and anger around a recent lost love is all wrapped up in my sadness at watching my mother die a very slow and scary death. My own fears of being self-employed, spending thousands of dollars on my art and writing careers, with not enough money coming back in right now from sales and jobs, compounds my concerns around managing Mary's money and making sure there is plenty there, just in case she lives another couple, three years or more. My own loneliness with having no one to share my bed mixes with my sadness at losing this sweet kind mother I've had for the past few months. But at the same time as all of this fury of emotions fills me, day in and day out, I feel this incredible gratitude. I have money to draw from, for Mom, for me and for some other good folk in my life. I have real friends who care about me and are really there for me, as I go through all of this. I'm there for them as they go through their own health scares, heartaches, job insecurities, and family crises, from Northern California to Upstate New York. And I have this strong faith that this will eventually end, be it my Mom's long suffering or my own grief or my friends' fears. Even though it's not OK, not even close to being OK, we'll all be OK, even in Death.

"...I want my Momma. I want my Momma. I want my Momma...."

"I want my Momma too," I say to Mary. I chuckle. That's not going to happen. I'm Mary's parent now, not she mine. And I'm happy to be your Mother, Mary. And maybe, just maybe, your Momma, my grandmother Nannie, will cross over from the other side and lend us a hand.

DISCOMBOBULATED

TUCSON, ARIZONA • CHRISTMAS, 2009

Got the call from Cousin Becky around nine p.m. on Christmas Eve, while having good talk and good coffee with Craig at Safehouse. Seems Aunt Virginia, my mother's oldest sister who also lives in Tucson, had a massive seizure earlier in the day. Virginia now can't eat, can't swallow, can't see, maybe can't hear. Her gaze is fixed. She's in a coma. She'll be dead within one to three days, say the nurses. She's home, not at a hospital. I told Becky I'll bring Mary by on the day after Christmas to see her sister.

"I'll roll the dice that Virginia lives until then," I told her. My intuition tells me she will. I also know from watching Dad die, that people often fight for life to the bitter end.

I swung by on Christmas Morning to visit Virginia on my way to Mary's, not for any nobler reason than to just get the lay of the land, to see just how bad Virginia looked. She looked pretty awful, her eyes wide open and unblinking, the death rattle in full force, each breath literally could be her last, her body in the throws. She will be dead soon. Could be a minute, could be a week.

Later, I'm sitting with Mary and her unwrapped Christmas presents of dresses and chocolate, when I give her the news. I ask her if she wants to go say goodbye to her sister.

"Well, of course I do!" she says, but her face reveals she has many questions. I've gotten pretty good at reading Mary's face.

"Now, I have to tell you Mom. This is going to hurt. Physically. Getting you in and out the car is going to be a bit painful. And you probably won't remember this house very well, and you'll be discombobulated when you get back. There could be a price to pay. Do you still want to go?" I ask.

Mary thinks for a bit, but not too long. Softly, she says "Yes."

Second day of Christmas and we're off in Mary's Buick La Sabre, which is now my car. She talks about how she drove this car just last week and that she's a good driver. I let it go. The staff dressed Mary in a very pretty red and green Holiday dress and we have spare blankets and diapers galore. In the trunk is a travel wheelchair, not the one hospice has provided for my mother's care, with its very high back. Her inability to hold up her head and steady herself could be a major issue on this short little trip.

"Mom, they know we are coming."

"That's good."

"Virginia won't be able to see you but she'll probably be able to hear you."

"I hope so."

I phone her brother Courtney as I drive. I hand the phone to Mary. They have a brief conversation. Gist is he'll find a way to make it to the funeral from Silver City, New Mexico. This seems to make Mary happy. She'll forget she talked with him in an hour, but the call makes her smile. All Mary has, these days, is the Here and Now, with no emotional context to anything in the past, and no hope for anything pleasant in her future. But it doesn't matter. Present Happiness is where it's at with her, and that's OK. Within thirty minutes of my returning her to her care home, she'll be complaining to the staff that I never come and see her, but that's all right as well. I have pretty good boundaries, and I don't take it personal. I know what I do and I know what I don't. I have no attachment to getting any approval from my mother at this point. Frankly, not now, not for decades.

We arrive at Freedom Inn, where Virginia lives in the much higher rent district of the Foothills than where my mother lives (even though Mary isn't in a bad part of town by any stretch.) I pretty much lift Mary's dead-weight out of the car and into her chair. Sure glad I still have some upper body strength. Summer surfing must have helped.

"Lift your feet, Mom." She does and off we go. [We could put footrests on the wheelchair for her, but she seems to quite enjoy lifting her feet as I push her. Gives her the illusion that she's doing something to propel herself along.]

Freedom Inn isn't that much different from The Santa Catalina Villas, the assisted living/independent living place Mom lived where she first moved to Tucson. Actually, I think they are owned by the same company. We roll past the dining hall, where lunch is being served. Men and women in wheelchairs, some with their own caregiver, some not. Up the elevator to Virginia's floor. Push Mary down the long hall, the whole place quiet as a tomb. I hate cliches but this place is a tomb, or rather the waiting room for one.

We enter Virginia's apartment. There's Becky, strong and in charge, in a good way. There's a caregiver and a nurse too. There's cousin Sally, eyes puffy from crying. Becky, a devout atheist; Sally, a big time born-again Christian; their deceased father Len, an Air Force chaplain, and Virginia, Southern Belle, a cradle-to-grave Episcopalian.

Welcome to the rich side of my family.

Too bad Mom hadn't met Dad before her father Earl died, for maybe the Jenks would have gotten some of that old Virginia property that partly propelled the Edmonds into the rich people they became later in life. All we got was my mother's Mom, Nannie, after she had lost everything. But I loved having Nannie in our house when I was little. Nannie was the only one who didn't have some weird opinion about my small presence in the home. [Mary didn't really know how to relate to children, being the narcissist she was. Dad didn't really want to have kids in the first place, and he made that clear to me by spending all his free time in the basement or in the garage. Little Stu was not invited. And Pamela seemingly hated me from the second I drew breath. That only changed after I moved Mom out to Tucson, a year and a half ago, and took Mary out of my sister's time zone and out of her hair.]

Becky moves a chair so Mary can be wheeled closer to her sister's deathbed. She leaves the room, and shuts the door. Nice of her to offer privacy but it's not really necessary. Mary doesn't feel any embarrassment now. Shame was never a big part of Mom's emotional makeup anyway and she doesn't really have much depth of feeling at all these days. She does have emotions, but it's more like those of a five year old girl, unhappy that she doesn't get what she wants sometimes, sad that something gets lost, happy when something delights her, and then it all quickly fades away into the next experience. There isn't much emotional memory, and that is a huge blessing.

The bedroom's loud now with the sound of a oxygen ventilator that's connected to Virginia's nose. Also a blessing for I can no longer hear the deep resonance of Virginia's heavy breathing and death rattle, like I did on Christmas Day.

"Hey Virginia, this is Stu." Her eyes now fixed to the right, the light that was just barely there yesterday, close to completely gone. Her body's alive and her soul's still there but not much more.

"I've brought your sister Mary so she can say goodbye."

I grab Virginia's hand to hold but it's limp. Yesterday, there was life. Today, just cold flesh.

"Well, it's Virginia," says my Mom. "It looks just like you!"

"Your hair looks so nice, Virginia. You always had nice hair."

Virginia's hair is just hair. Not good or bad. It's hard to miss those eyes.

"Well... I love you, Virginia."

And that was it. Mary and I silently look at her sister, and don't speak for a while. I look at Mary's face. It isn't sad, or glad, or anything. Just kind of blank and expressionless. I chuckle. My face probably looks close to that too, but mine's from being really tired these days. Mary's is from just not having enough active brain cells.

I wheel her out of Virginia's bedroom and we say our goodbyes. Mary comments on how thin Becky is. She says how good it is to see Sally, as we met up with her at the front door of the place. I pick Mom up, placed her in the front seat, wheelchair in the trunk and off we go, back to Crossroads.

We stop and get a Vanilla milkshake from a McDonald's drive-thru, and within twenty minutes we are on the residential street that leads to her place. We drive up to her home for the last year, and she looks at it as if she's never seen it before. Park and unload and back inside. We say hello to the residents who include happy Down's Syndrome young adults, smiling white haired old ladies in wheelchairs, grumpy old demented men who spout nonsense, and pouty elderly women who wear permanent frowns. The caregiver (a delightful woman from Thailand) and I agree that we should put Mary to bed. As I wheel Mary toward her room, she demands to go back to the kitchen and living room where most of the residents are hanging out.

"I want to see them," she says.

"OK," I say.

"Hello, everyone," she announces, after we return to the residents.

No one says anything to Mary. A pretty white haired lady smiles at Mom, but it's no way near enough. Mary wants attention and there is none coming her way. She pouts.

I take her back to her room and put her to bed. She hasn't brought up Virginia since we left her place. That doesn't exist anymore and sadly, neither does this house.

"Back to your room that you've lived in for over a year," I say, "And there's your dresser, and there are the pictures of me and Annie and Susie. And that's me there," pointing to two pictures, one, Stu in a kilt, the other, Stu on a surf board. "And there's Annie," of her at an Art opening, "And there's Susie," taken of her at sunset, on a California cliff that overlooked the Pacific Ocean.

Mary hears me talking and is vaguely looking at the pictures but I can see anxiety on her face.

She doesn't remember this room. She doesn't remember this house. She doesn't remember the people.

This is the price I knew we would pay for leaving the house. But knowing this didn't make visiting her dying sister the wrong choice. And it wasn't the right choice, because Mary needed to say goodbye to Virginia. She didn't need to do that. She and Virginia barely get along. There is no moral imperative that these two sisters see each other one last time. Yet there is nothing wrong with Mary going to Virginia's deathbed, even if it means Mom will be severely discombobulated for a few days.

It was the right thing to do, simply because Mary wanted to do it.

If I'm dying and I want to go on the roof of my house and watch a sunset, find a ladder. Don't argue with me. Don't say it won't be good for me, or it's foolish. Just find a goddamn ladder and get me up there, so I can have the warm Sun on my face, one last time. And if I ask to go up again the next day, do it. Understand? Listen to the dying. They will always tell you what they want, and if it's different from what you want, that's just too damn bad!

Cowboy up, boys and girls. Cowboy up.

MR. LET-US-PRAY

TUCSON, ARIZONA • WINTER, 2010

Another grumpy day for Mom. She isn't making much sense but she continues to talk and talk and talk. One thing for sure I can tell you; she isn't happy. No, her sister dying last week isn't why she's unhappy. They didn't much get along. She's frankly looking forward to Virginia's funeral for she gets to leave Crossroads for a few hours and I'm sure she'll like all the attention. No, she's having one of those days where she knows what's happening to her, that she's living in a very nice house with very good food and a very sweet staff, surrounded by other people who are dying of dementia or worse, and she can't escape it except through death. It's just pissing her off today. Who would blame her? Not I.

I'm getting ready to leave Crossroads, when the Catholic Lay Couple arrive. They come twice a week to say the Lord's Prayer over the clients. I frankly don't much like them.

A few months back, we thought Mary was dying. I was sitting and talking with my mother while she drifted in and out of sleep in her bed. I was just getting something from her that I kind of understood, when Mr. Catholic Layman entered her room.

"Could you give us a couple of minutes?" I asked, "And then you can pray with her."

He smiled down at me in my chair and ignored my request, pushing past me toward my mother and beginning to talk with her.

"Hello, sweetheart," he said, "We're here to pray with you."

What the fuck?

I thought of confronting him right then and there, but instead I said a silent prayer and the answer came back, 'Not now.'

Ok, I thought. But next time that son of a bitch decides that he and God are more important than me, I will pull him aside and say sometime to the effect of:

"Listen, pal. I appreciate you coming and visiting with my mother, but you blew me off a while ago when I asked you nicely, to give my mother and I some time. So right now, listen very closely. When I'm here, I trump God. I trump you. I fucking trump everyone in the house. Capiche? If I ask you to wait, you wait. If I ask you to leave, you leave. If ask you to do a fucking dance, you dance a fucking jig. Comprende, padre?"

I'm sure he'll give me a pious smile, but I'll continue to look him square in the eye and I'll end with a little smile of my own, my crazy-motherfucker-smile, and I'll say:

"Do we have an understanding?"

If he ignores me, I'll gently but firmly grab his arm and say again:

"Do you understand me?"

He will then.

Let's hope it doesn't come to this. I'm a good guy but I can be a real bastard when it's called for.

Today, it's not called for. I'm getting ready to leave anyway.

I say hello to Mr. and Mrs. Catholic Laypeople. They barely acknowledge my presence. Jerks.

Mr. Catholic walks up to my mother, who's sitting on a sofa in the living room, watching cartoons.

"Well, hello sweetie, how are you doing?"

Her name's Mary and she isn't your sweetie.

Mom looks up at him as he approaches her and says loudly, with matter-of-fact disdain in her voice:

"LOOK HERE. IT'S MISTER LET-US-PRAY!"

Goes completely over his head.

"Mom, I'm going to go. I'll see you tomorrow."

I give her a kiss and start to leave the house. As soon as I close the front door behind me, I can't hold it in any longer. I loudly guffaw all the way to the car.

VIRGINIA'S FUNERAL

TUCSON, ARIZONA • WINTER, 2010

Mary sits in a pew, looking at the church bulletin, at her sister's face with its birth and death dates under it, and it hits her, as if she just heard about Virginia's death for the first time. She starts to cry hard.

"Stop it, Mary. Stop it," she says to herself.

"It's OK to cry, Mom," I whisper to her. "It's really quite sad. It's OK to miss your sister."

"I don't want to cry. Stop it, Mary," she says, scolding herself.

Mom, even when she was in her right mind, would never had been described as being touchy-feely. Histrionic? Yes. Honest expression of emotion? No.

I touch Mary's arm, and don't say anything else. I'm just there.

Others are there too. Virginia's two daughters. A cousin-once-removed that I've met once before. Various members of the congregation at Grace St. Paul's Episcopal Church.

And my mother's only brother, Courtney.

I was talking to Craig on my cell on the way to the church today.

"I'm praying I keep my powder dry today. I'm praying to not rise to the bait if Courtney throws out some chum," I said.

We both chuckle but Craig knows that it could turn ugly, if I lose my shit.

You see, Courtney and I had words a couple of months ago. The last time I visited him in New Mexico, I told him to shut the fuck up. (I got tired of his racist proclamations. What can I say? Some days I'm good. Some days I'm bad. That day both Courtney and I were bad.)

Fifteen minutes have passed. Mary has forgotten why she's here. Then she looks at her bulletin again and realizes again, that Virginia is dead and gone. Again. She cries like she just heard the news, even though her sister has been dead for ten days.

"Stop it, Mary, Stop it!" she says loud enough for me and others to hear.

"It's OK, Mom. It's OK to cry," I whisper.

Then the shade of her dementia comes down again, and she's looking around the church like a little girl.

"This is a nice building," she says, not knowing she's sat in this sanctuary, this Episcopal Church, dozens of times over the last twenty years.

"Yes, it is a very nice church," I say.

An elder man approaches the alter and begins to sing The Lord's Prayer a cappella. Quite lovely. Then his solo becomes a duet with Mary kinda sorta singing along. She's not even close to the right key, and who knows what words she is singing, but she looks happy. Like a small child who hasn't learned what's the right and wrong behavior for church. She belts out a song. I don't touch her for I don't want her to stop. Her sister's dead and it's her funeral as much as any other family members. Sing on, Mary Jenks.

I do my eulogy of Virginia. (I did Len's and Dad's and now Virginia's. The family knows I can write and that's a nice thing. And it lets them off the hook I suppose from a public display of emotion. I have no problem talking through tears at the pulpit. It's who I am. Hell, I should start charging.) I tell a few stories about my aunt. I say that I'll miss her but I really won't, for we weren't that close. But I do cry as I say those words for I'm sad watching my mother be so sad, so confused, so self-critical on a day when she should feel any expression of grief is appropriate.

Father McBride gives a nice homily. Communion's fine. I wave my wafer over the cup like I've done for 25 years since I stopped drinking alcohol. I return to my seat and push Mary's wheelchair back to our place on the far left aisle of the second row of pews. Half the congregation passes us as they leave the communion rail. A woman in a wide hat who I don't know from Adam stops to say hello to Mom.

"So sorry for your loss," says The Hat Lady.

"Why, thank you," says Mom, appearing not quite certain what the woman is talking about.

"Did you ever marry?" asks the woman.

Oh, this ought to me good.

"Yes, I did."

"Did you have any children?"

What am I lady! Chopped Liver?

"Yes," says Mary. "I have three children."

Hmm. There's Pamela and I. Wonder who the third child is. Something you haven't told me, Mom? Probably Annie. 'You're the daughter I never had,' she would say to Annie, years ago when she was getting sick and tired of her own daughter.

"God bless you," says The Hat Lady.

"Thank you," says my mother.

Christ.

After the service, there is a small reception. Jessica, the nurse from Crossroads, who brought Mary to the service, wheels her over to the parish hall. I walk beside Mom, hugging a number of my church friends as we make our way over. I'm very happy to have so many friends. They all say my eulogy was wonderful. I thank them, and hug them a second time.

As I make my way over to the reception, I notice Courtney sitting in his wheel chair on the sidewalk away from the church. My two cousins, Becky and Sally, Sally's husband, Jim and Becky's son, Scott encircle Courtney and seem to be talking in earnest with him. I promised my sister I'd say hello to Courtney and this is as good a time as any.

"Hey Courtney. How you doing?" I don't wait for an answer. "Pamela sends her love and wanted me to tell you that she loves the gold piece of jewelry that you gave her many years ago that you bought in Saudi Arabia."

"Is that right?" he says with a smile on his face. Good. He's trying to be nice to me. I'm smiling too. It's a fake smile but sometimes you've got to be a phony just to get along.

"Yep. She wears it around her neck to this day. You coming to the reception?

"No. I'm going to stay here," says Courtney.

That's odd.

"Ok. Well, have a safe journey back to Silver City."

"Thank you," he says, his smile fading a bit.

"Take care," I say, weakly smiling myself, and then I walk back to the parish hall.

What was that all about?

I found out later at dinner with my cousins that Courtney had absolutely refused to come over to the parish hall. That he had basically been his usual weird-ass, pain-in-the-neck self since he entered the church.

"I don't know if I'm going to be welcome here!" he loudly proclaimed as he arrived, to all the priests at the front door of the church.

"You can just dig a hole and throw me in the ground when I die. Don't fuss over me!" I heard him say that myself, during the Passing of the Peace. Didn't surprise me at the time. He's been saying that phrase since I as a kid.

What I didn't know until dinner was this:

As Scott pushed Courtney out of the church after the funeral and began to steer toward the parish hall, Courtney planted his feet on the ground and stopped his progress.

"I'm not going to go over there. Push me to the sidewalk," said my uncle. "Go ahead, dear and get yourself something to eat," he said to his nurse who had driven him over from New Mexico. "I'll be here and then we can go home."

Scott, Becky and Sally pleaded with him to come inside. Tried for at least fifteen minutes to convince him to go to the reception but he would have none of it. They even brought him some water but he was firm and resolute.

"I'm staying right here."

When asked for a reason, he gave none.

At dinner that night, my cousins who knew Courtney were not surprised, nor I, but Scott and his wife who didn't know their great-uncle that well, were amused but shocked. I sat at the elegant table at The Arizona Inn, with my Buffalo Filet in front of me, cut a piece, placed it in my mouth, moaned with delight, and just shock my head and smiled. I wondered for a moment if Courtney hadn't come into the parish hall because of our recent confrontation, but then remembered that this behavior of his was the norm, not the exception. Courtney simply always does what Courtney wants to do. Been that way forever. And this afternoon, he just didn't want to go into the parish hall. Even he probably didn't know why.

Driving home from The Arizona Inn, I think back on the day. Mary had a good time at the reception. She got a lot of attention and I'm happy for that, but she was so judgmental of her own sadness. Alas, her inner criticism of her own grieving hurt her more than the tears ever will. It's been that way for years, long before she got sick.

I take Swan Road north toward home. I chuckle to myself, thinking about Mary's best line of the day. Mom may be dying but she can still turn a phrase.

Jessica was packing Mom up in Grace's parish hall, getting ready to wheel Mary to the car when Mom said loudly for all to hear:

"Well, I sure don't want to do THAT again, anytime soon!"

I smile. I love you, Mom.

I look out the windshield and see the glow of Finger Rock, lit by the city lights behind me. I'm almost home.

MARY 4.0

TUCSON, ARIZONA • WINTER, 2010

Mom has rebooted again, but without the Microsoft Updates. More like a hard reinstall of all the old softwares. All the sweetness of the past few months is gone. All her attentiveness and compassion for her housemates has left. All of her kind motherly love for me is no more. It's like the Good Mother I've had for the past three months never existed. We're back to the selfish, self-centered woman I've been dealing with for the past 55 years. Only difference is she can't remember what happened three minutes ago. But her angry pronouncements that 'Nobody ever visits me.' 'I hate this room.' 'The people here are awful,' and 'I thought you would never come to see me.' are now mixed with continuous chatter, most of it unbelievably hard to follow, yet clearly spoken:

"I went out on the town and then they dropped something."

"He was here but then he left."

"He just drove by. That was him."

"We sure had a something, I tell you."

"Mom, I can't understand a thing you are saying," I say.

"I'll try harder," she says.

"Trying's not going to help, Mom."

"I went out this morning and we drove to some place."

"Mom, you haven't left this house for six months and that was when you were in the hospital."

"Abcdefghijklmnop"

That's new.

"Will I ever buy a new car?" she asks.

"No, you won't. You haven't driven a car in 14 months."

"I haven't?"

"No, Mom, you haven't"

"Are you sure?"

"I'm positive."

"I want to... That woman is terrible," responding to the voice of one of the caretakers in the hall.

"Mom, everyone here loves you." [The staff really does love Mary. Every other resident in the house is either mute or brain-impaired. Mary at least talks.]

"Why is it this way?" she asks.

I tell her for the 100th time. I don't mind telling her the truth. She used to like the truth, demanded it actually, and she felt happy to hear it. Hell if I know now.

"Mom, you are dying of dementia. It's that Brain Thing. Your body's deteriorating because of your Brain Thing. You can't drive, walk, write or go to the bathroom by yourself. The feeling on your right side is almost completely gone now. You can't remember things. And none of it is your fault. It's not your fault."

"I can try harder to remember."

"It won't matter, Mom. You don't have to remember. The staff and I are taking care of you and all the remembering. I know you aren't happy..."

"I'm not at all!"

"...I know, but I think if you can just accept what is happening to you a little, rather than fighting it, you might be a little happier."

"Puhh," she scoffs.

"You need to hear what I'm saying," she continues. "1, 2, 3. 1, 2, 3. Now you're upset."

"I am a little irritated," I say.

"Well, I just won't say anything," and she clams up like a petulant four-year-old.

I might have, in the past, filled this space with small talk. Not this afternoon. I let it hang. For a very long while. Close to a minute. I'm being petulant too. Two grownups acting like kids. She breaks the silence to ask the time.

"Quarter to Four. Dinner will be soon."

"Hummph."

I can't be around this any more today.

"Mom, I've got some work to do. Do you want to go back into the living room or stay here, in your bedroom?"

"I can't stay in the house anymore!"

"You going to have to, Mom."

"It's wrong!"

"Just accept it as best as you can."

I wheel Mary out to the rest of the house. It's dinner time. All the other residents but two are sitting at the dining room table. One woman, new to me, inches herself in her walker, ever so slowly toward her chair. I give her a hand and pull out the chair for her.

"Thank you," she says.

"You're welcome."

I return to Mary's wheelchair.

"Time to put you at the head of the table," I say.

"Good," she says.

Then she proclaims loudly to the everyone sitting around the table:

"This is my husband, Stuart!"

"No, Mom. I'm your son, Stu."

"We know that," says one of the residents, looking at me.

Mary gives me a look that says: 'Don't you correct me. I know what I'm talking about.'

I give her a kiss on the forehead and make my exit from Crossroads.

Driving away, I call Annie and give her the rundown of Mary's condition, and warn her what to possibly expect when she visits on Saturday.

"Oh, Jeez," she says.

"I know."

I've got to come up with my own whole new level of acceptance to this new situation with Mary. Accept that Sweet Mom is perhaps gone forever. And I'm pretty clear on this one thing. I won't be visiting Mary every day for a while. Four, five times a week, tops. At least for a while to protect my own sanity. Mary is already perpetually disappointed in me, whether I come every day, or never again. The compromise of every-other-day seems like the best way to go, at least for now.

Yet as Scarlet O'Hara said: 'Tomorrow is another day.' Then again, Scarlet stated that after Rhett had walked out on her. So who knows what part of Mary's brain will be with us tomorrow. Mary 5.0? Or perhaps a whole new operating system.

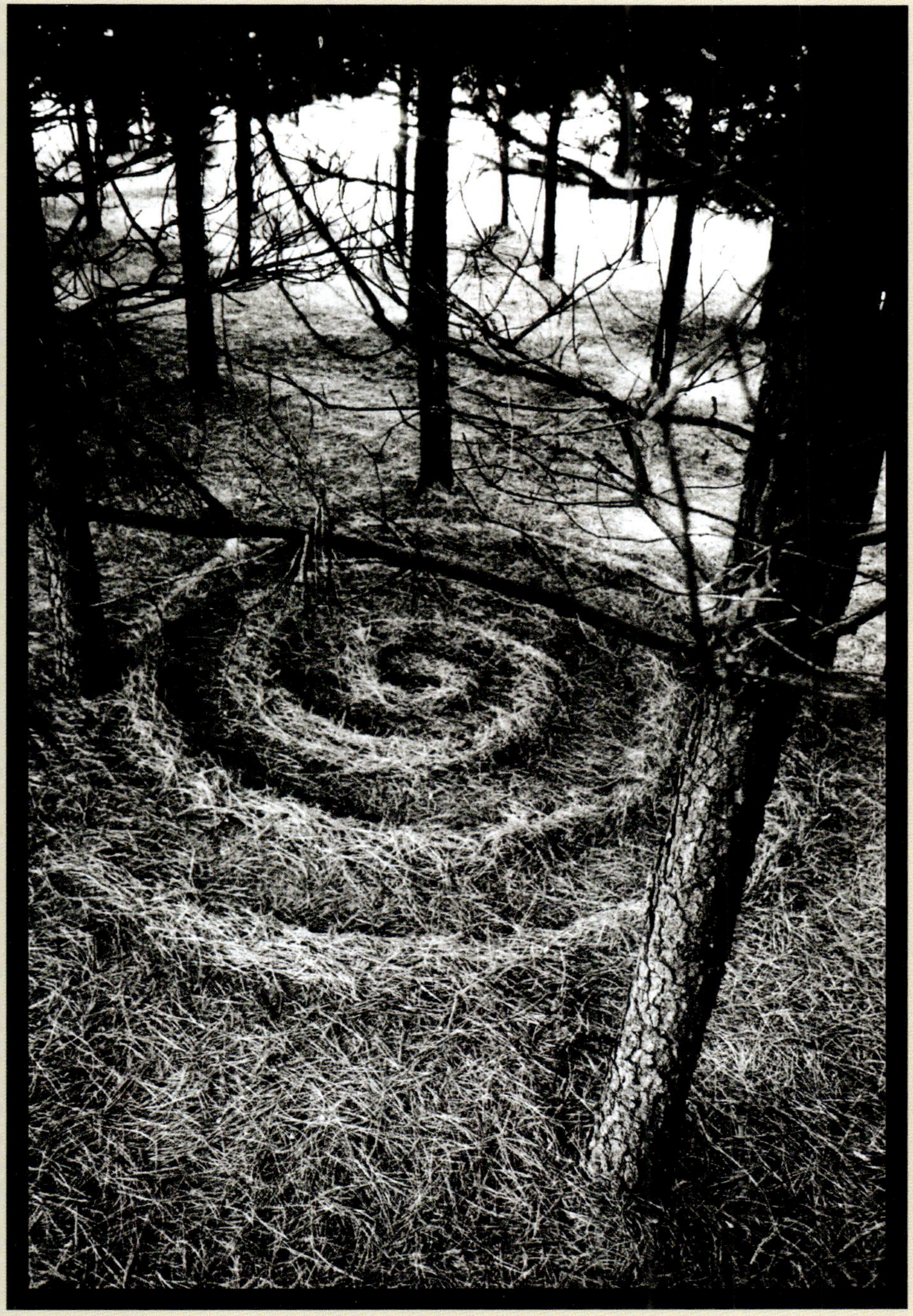

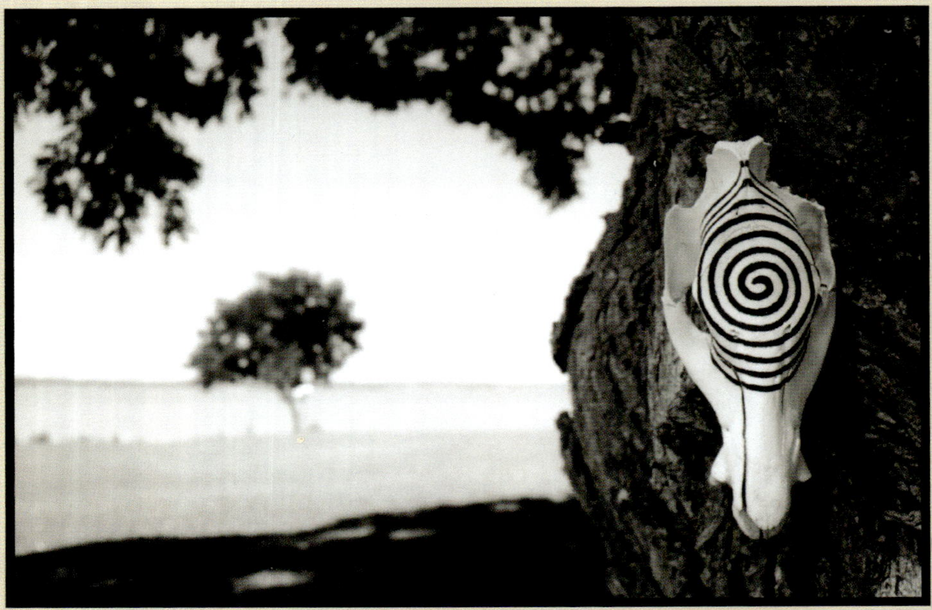

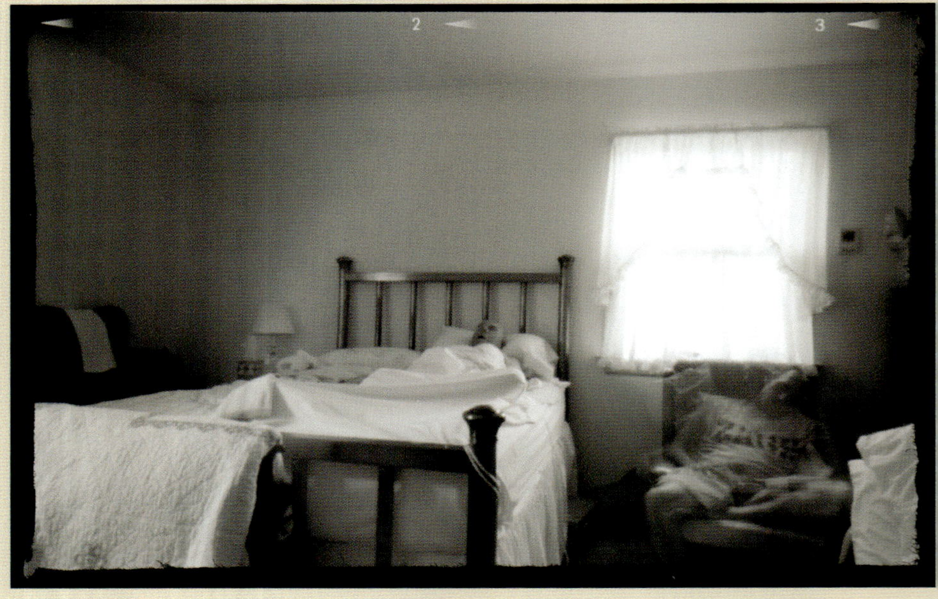

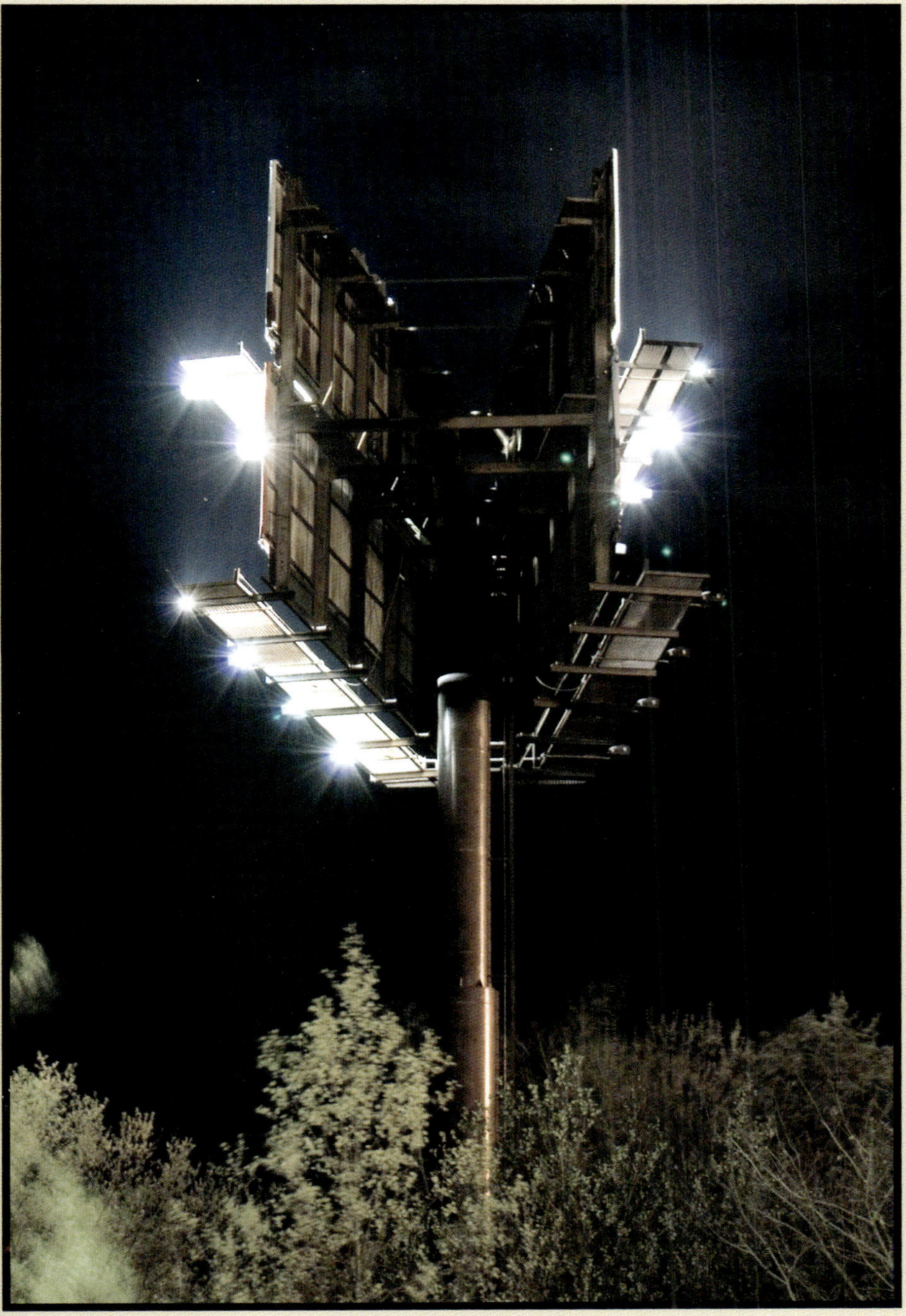

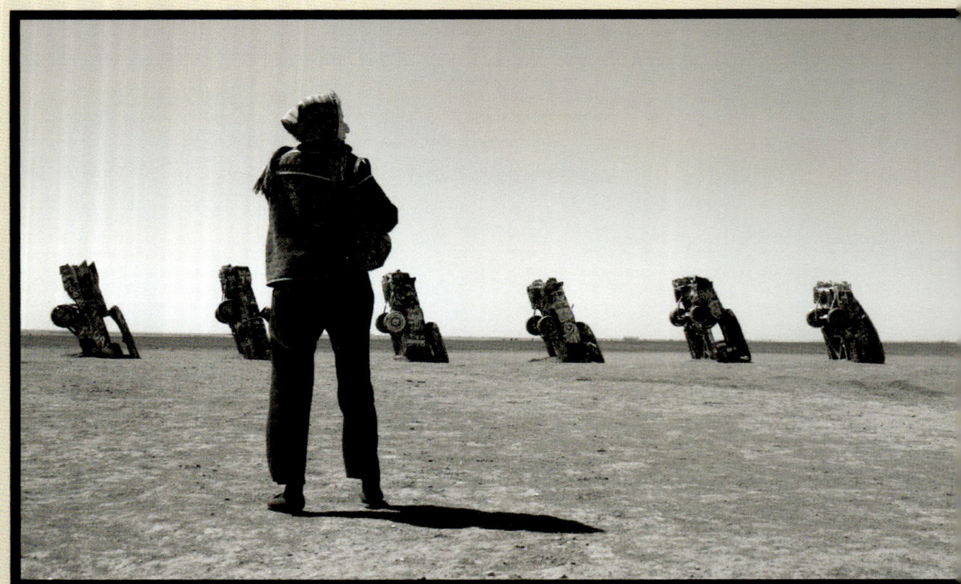

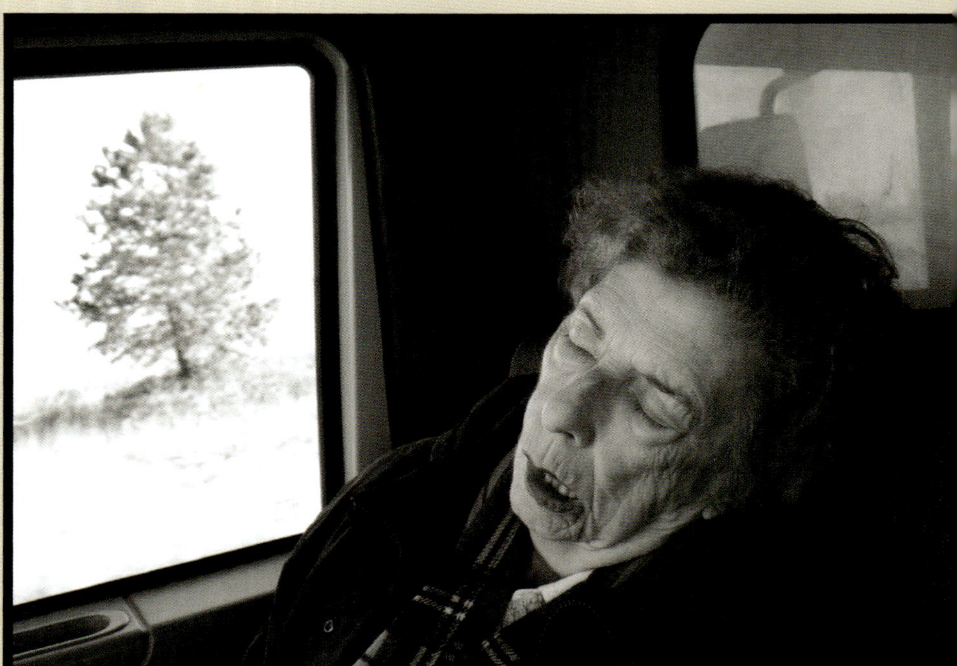

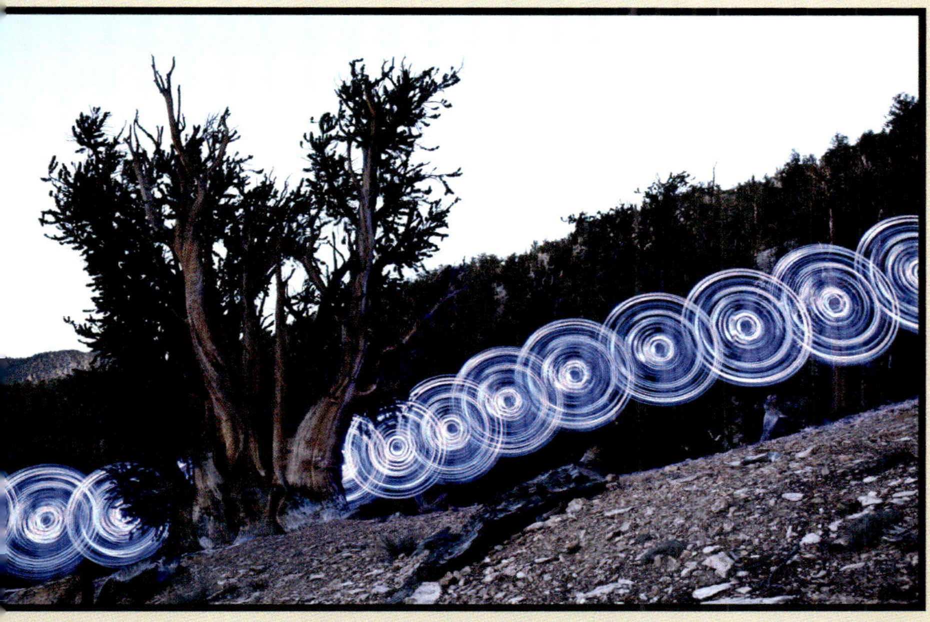

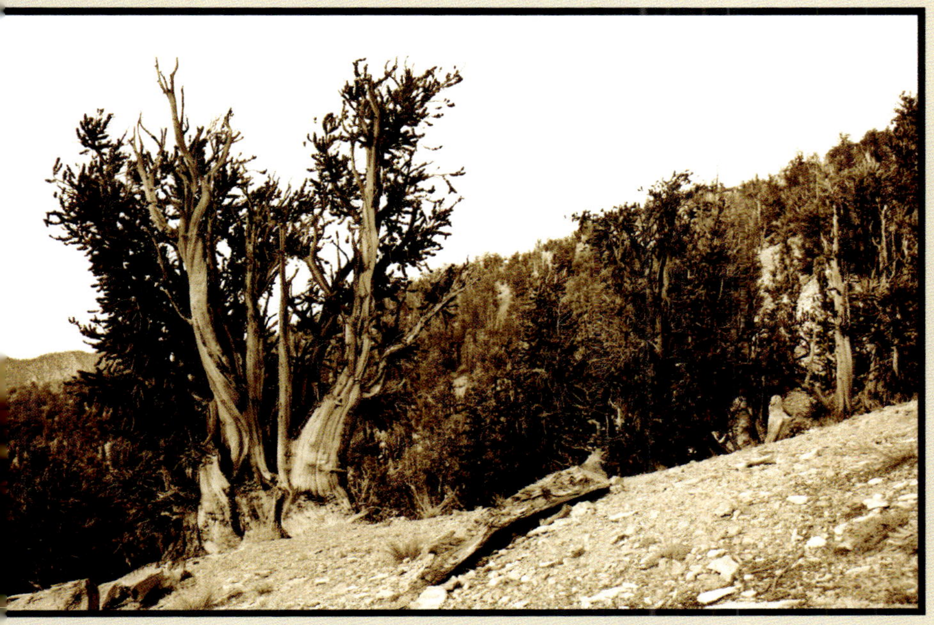

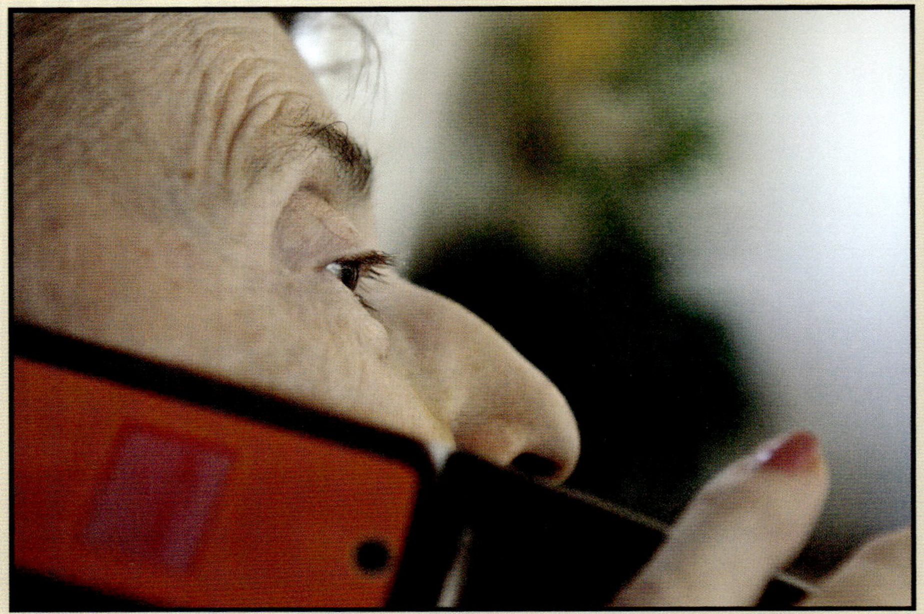

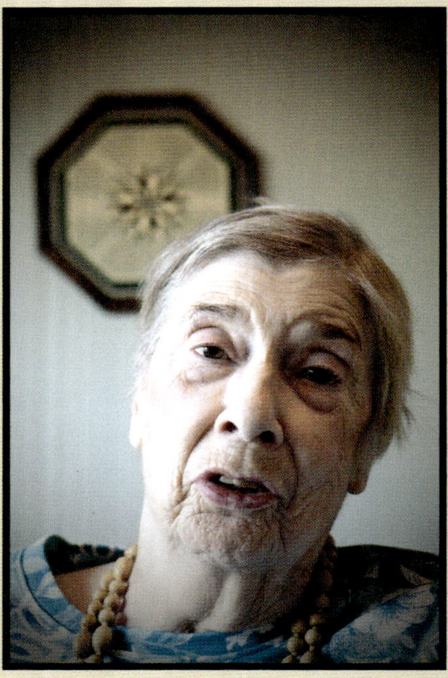

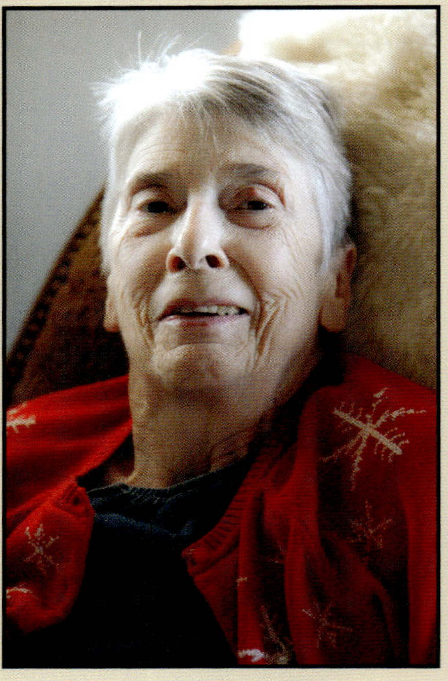

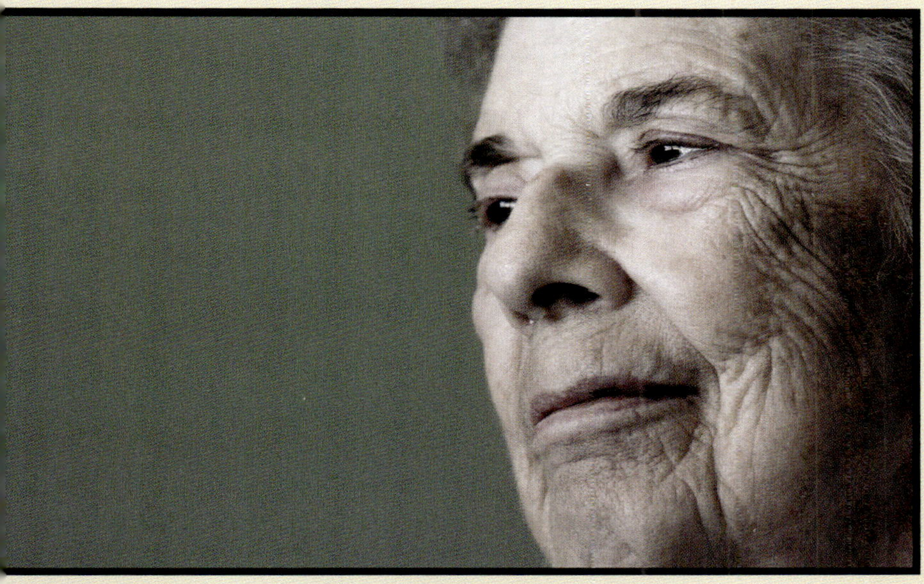

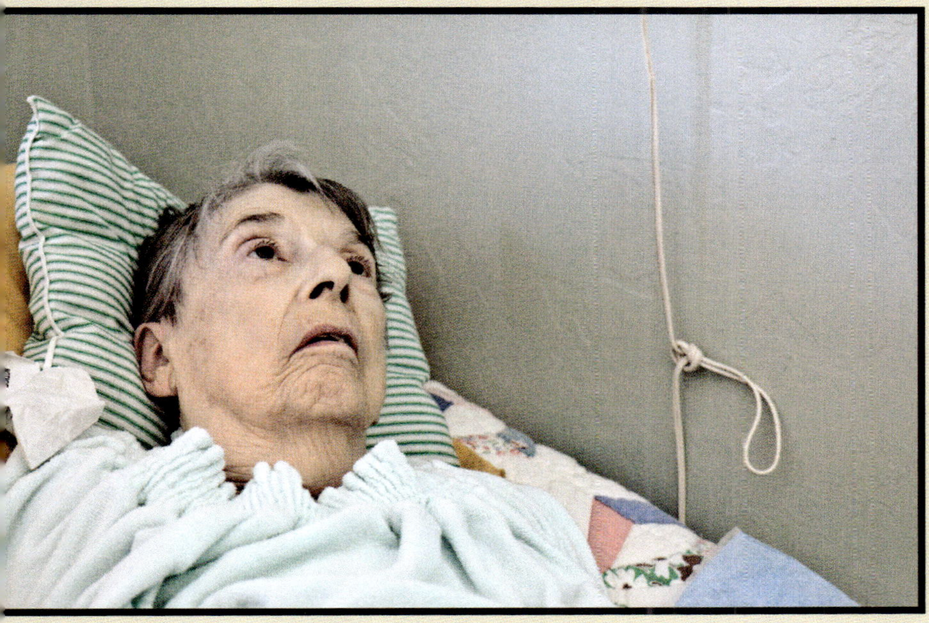

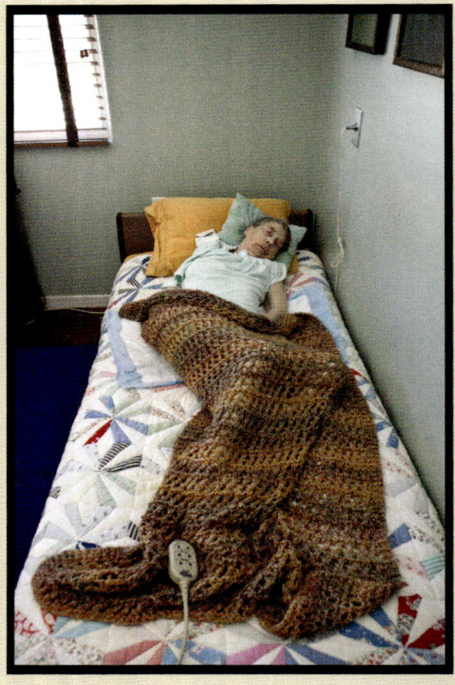

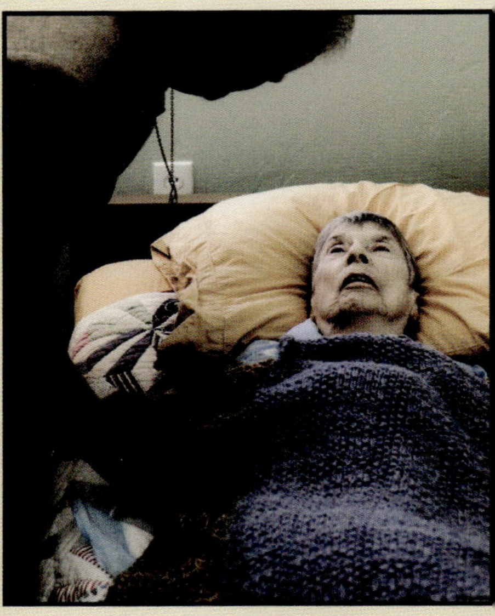

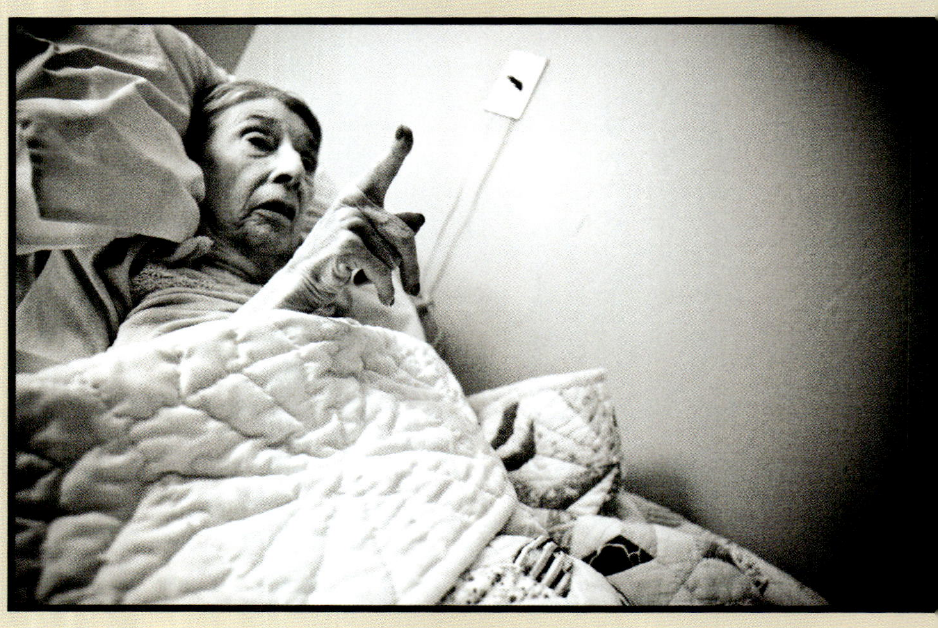

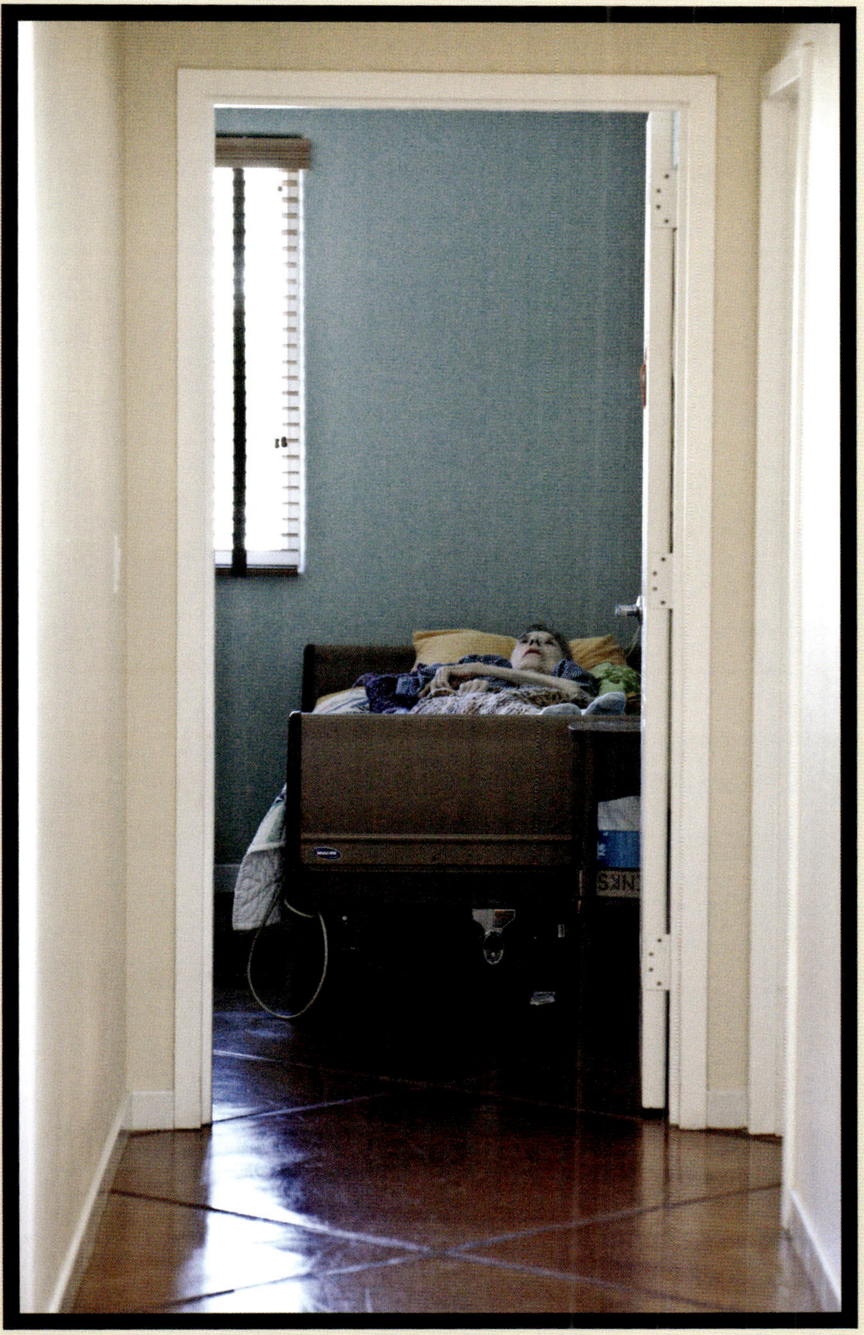

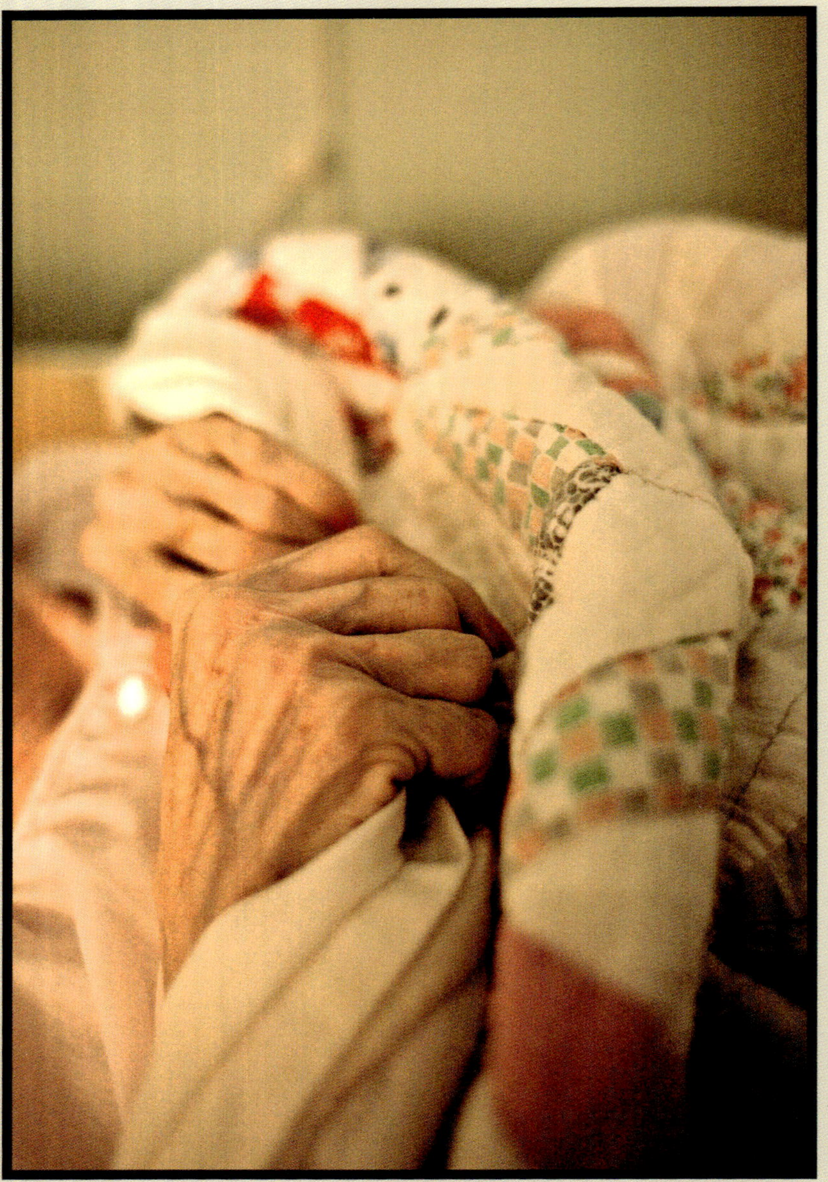

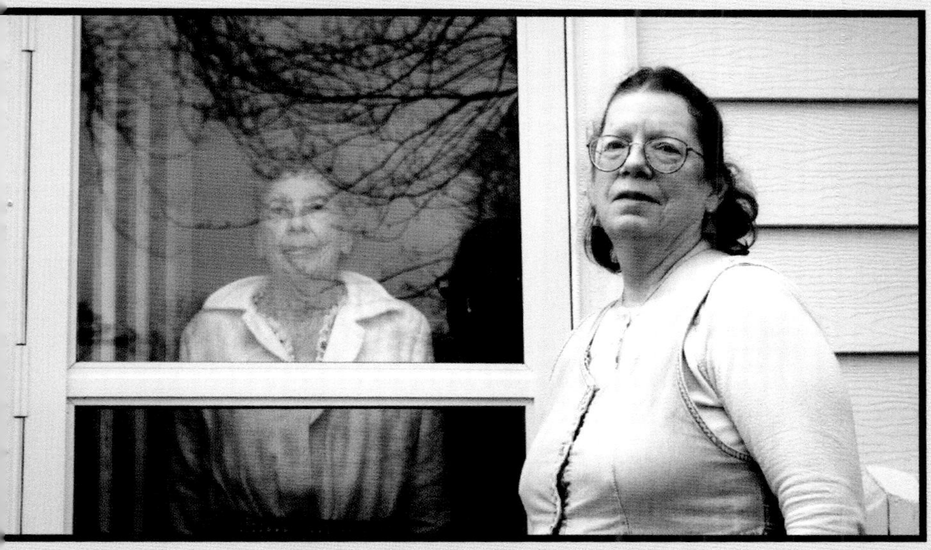

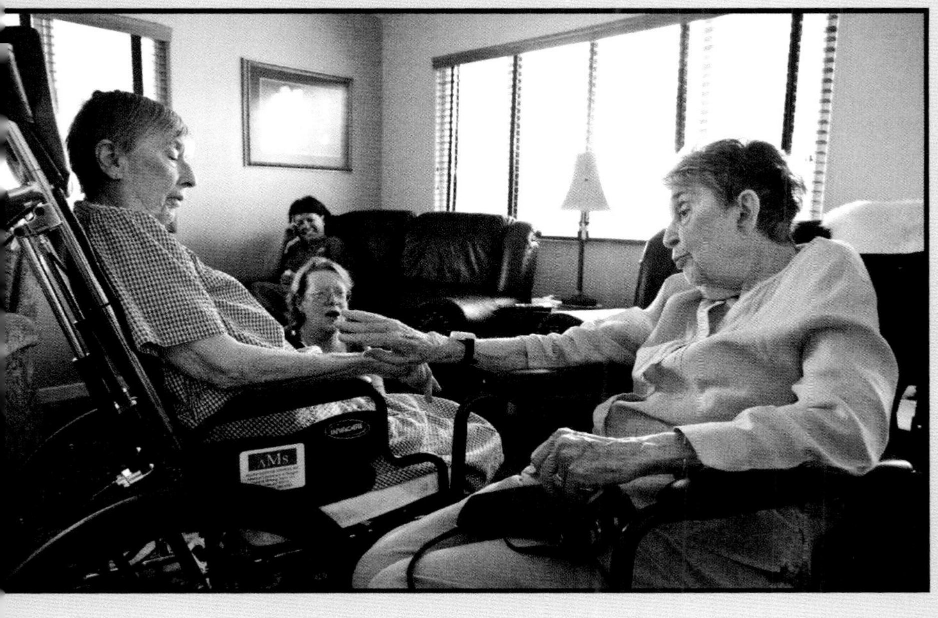

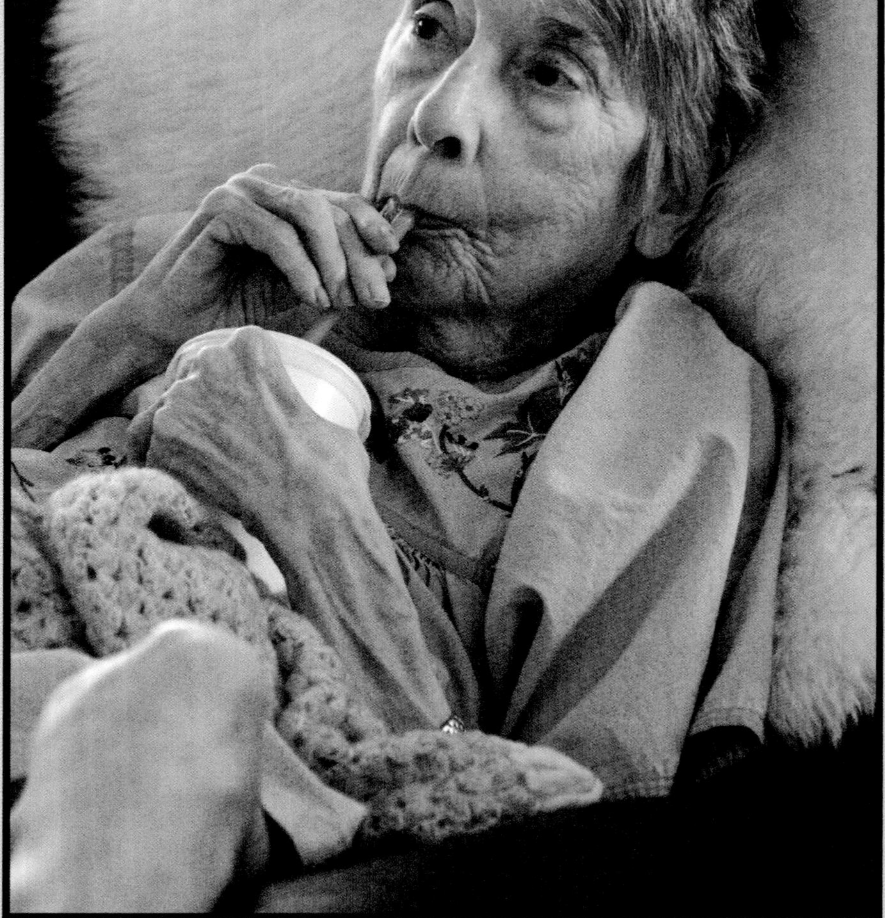

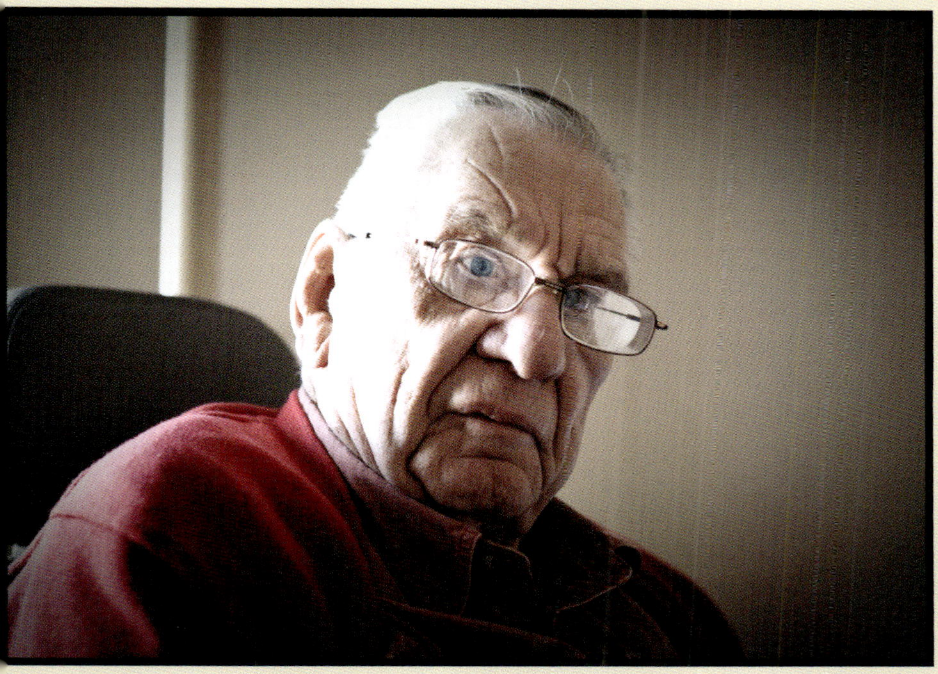

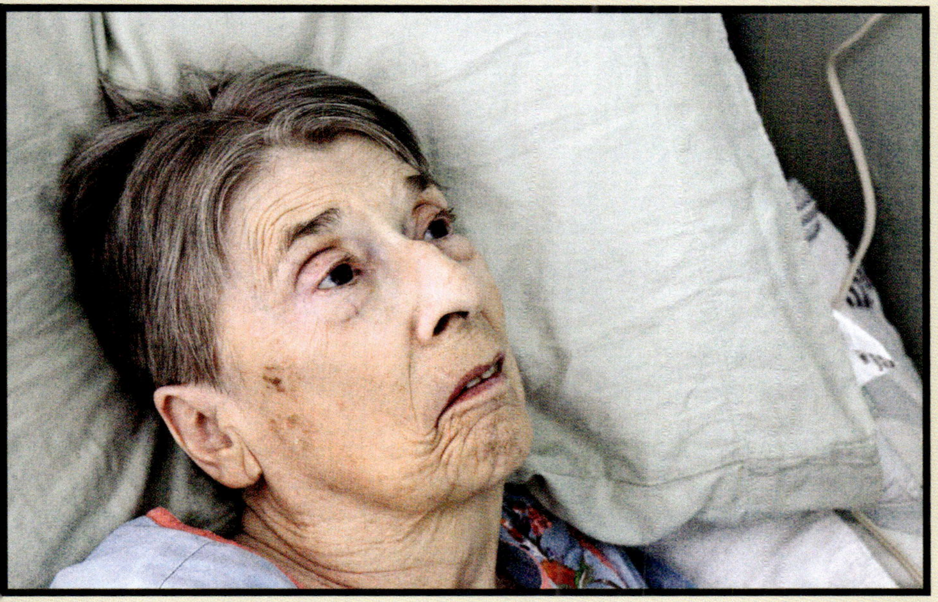

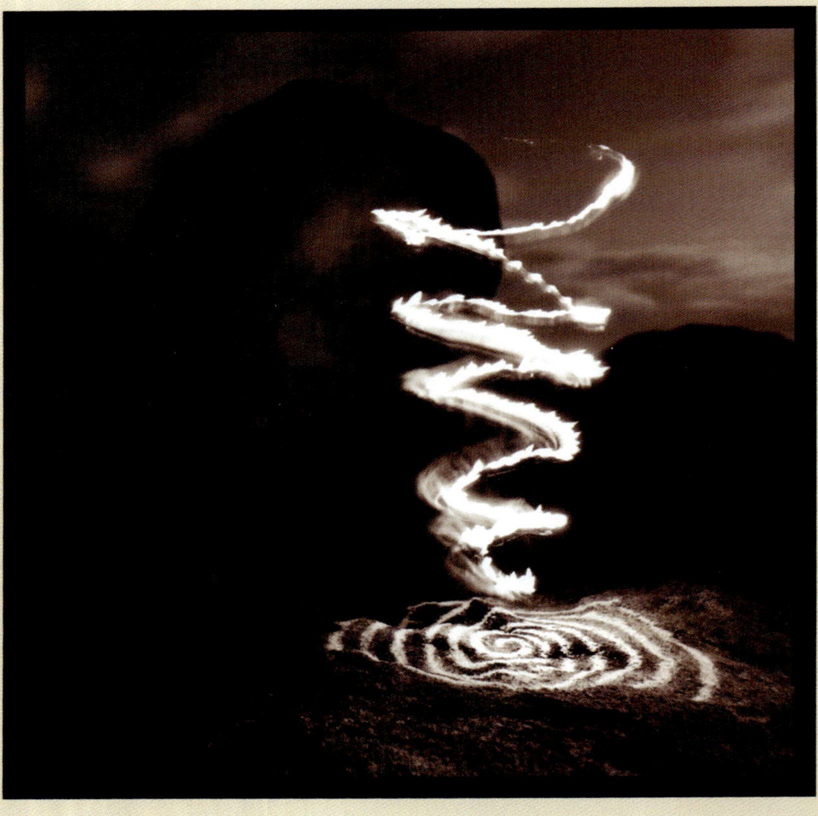

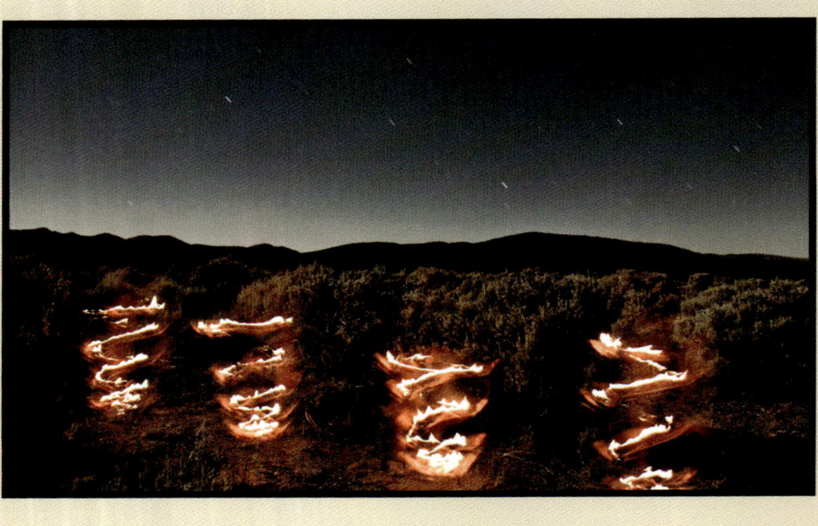

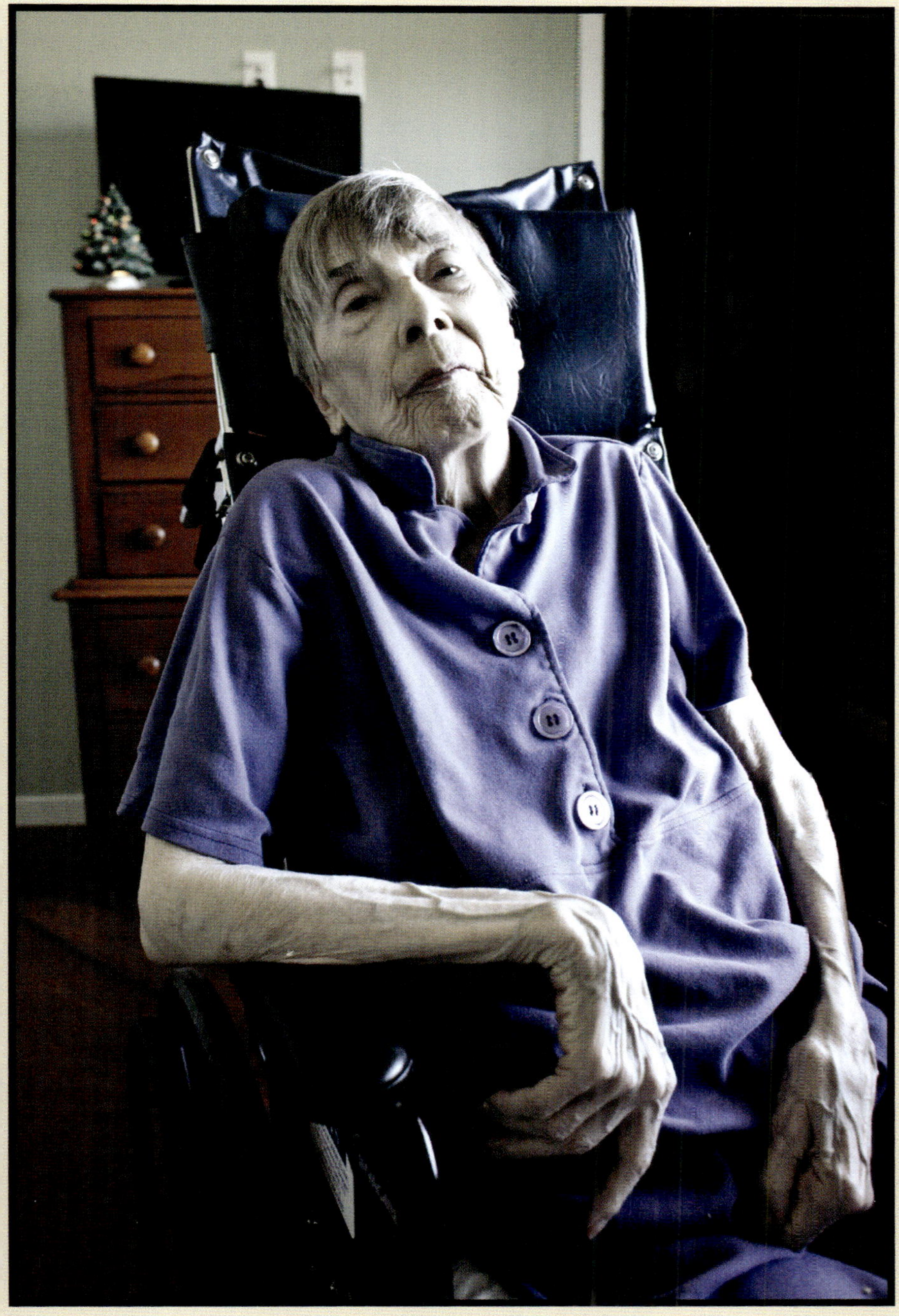

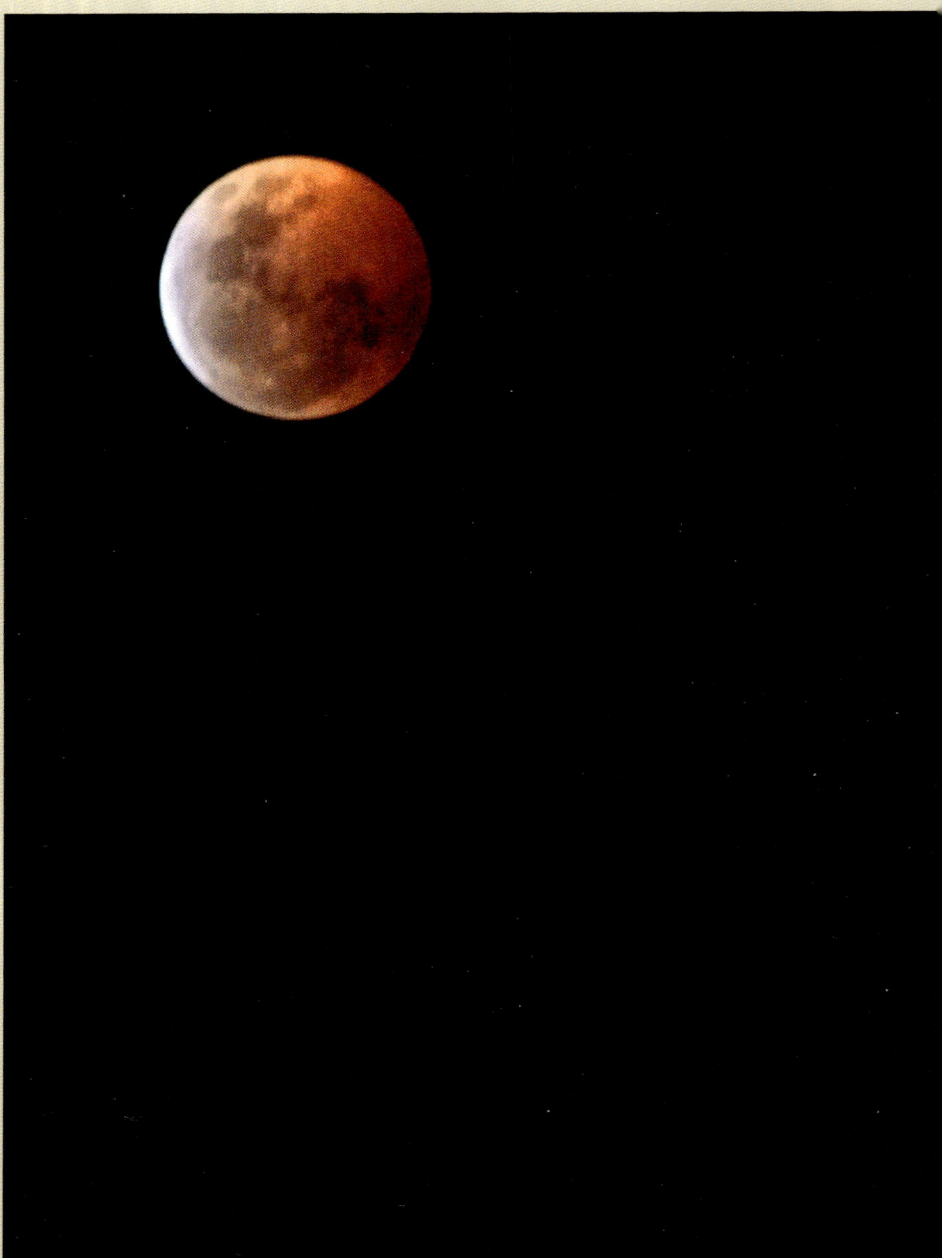

MARY'S ANXIOUS HANDS

TUCSON, ARIZONA • WINTER, 2010

I arrive and peer down the hall toward Mary's room. Door's half open. All I can see are her legs, half off the bed. I can hear her talking. I stop and talk with the nurse before walking down the hall.

"Is Mary with someone?"

"No, she by herself," says the Asian nurse. Her English isn't perfect, but she's a real sweetheart and a great caregiver. Really loves my Mom.

"Really? Is she just talking to herself?"

The nurse gives a sad look.

"Is this new or has she been doing this for a while?"

"A while."

I almost cry, right then and there. I can feel my eyes misting up. I stop the tears. I'll cry later.

"I didn't know."

"It just part of her disease," says the nurse.

"Yeah, I know. But I didn't know she was talking to herself."

"She talks a lot. She asks for you all the time." She isn't trying to shame me into anything. They know I visit Mary pretty much every day.

"Yea, that's what I hear," I smile weakly.

"Well, I'm going down to see her," I continue.

"Ok, Stu."

Mom's very happy to see me, but she's extra-special anxious today. Her voice is clear but the meaning of her words is not. Half are sentences about this and that. The other half are sentences that don't make a lick of sense. Then she says something that's very clear.

"Stu, I'm scared. Frightened. And you know I don't get scared," says Mom.

I also know feelings have never been Mary's middle name and that I had to do a ton of therapy years ago to get past all the devaluing of my feelings by her, and the rest of my family, when I was a child. Dad was the deep one. But distant. Very far away, even when he was in the same house as us.

"Really, Mom?"

"Yes. I don't know where I am. I just got here to this house today."

"No, Mom, you've been here 15 months and the staff loves you a lot."

That sentence about the staff caring for her and about her length of stay at Crossroads tends to be almost my daily salutation to Mary. 'Hi, Mom. You've been here x number of months and the nurses really love you a lot.' I draw a bit of Mary's life on her mental Etch-A-Sketch everyday and the dementia shakes it free every night. 'Dad's been dead x number of years.' 'You've had that cough for x number of years.', 'I'm Stu, not Courtney.' The other day, she started talking about me as if I wasn't there; about how Stu talks about her dying a lot, and she didn't like that very much. I mentioned to her that I was Stu and she got this funny look on her face. Like 'Oops'. Then ten minutes later she said that she wished she would die. I said, me too. The double bind doesn't bother me that much. I know it's not about me, nor ever has been.

"And I just sit here and I don't know what to do. I'm so scared."

No manipulation on her part. She's simply a scared 5-year-old girl in a dying 83-year-old woman's body.

"And I wish I could sleep."

"Now that, Mom," I say, "I can do something about. I'll talk with the nurses about giving you some more sleep medication."

"That would be so good."

I'll give Hospice a call on Monday. Maybe we can up her sedatives. Last time we did that, she slept a bunch, could hardly talk and had problems eating, but she wasn't freaking out all the time, and she had some peace of mind on Her Road to Death. Not now.

The goal is to have Mom die as easily as possible. It isn't to extend her life. Death with some grace is the object here, even though this may be at cross-purposes with some people and sometimes with Mary herself, but Mom isn't getting any better, and now she suffers more times than not. It makes me sad. It makes her afraid.

We all thought she was dying last Fall, but she rallied. I don't know who was more surprised, Mary or me. I used to call Mom's dying a mystery, being all spiritual and such. Now it's just a grind, a bad dream, a very slow exhalation followed by another unexpected deep breath.

I tell her about my day, or my night, or anything in my life. Just hearing my voice tends to calm her, even if she sometimes thinks I'm Dad, or her brother, or a kind stranger. More times than not though, she knows I'm Stu, her only son.

She's enjoying hearing about me winning at poker last night, and I mention Annie and the pretty flowers that Annie gave her, and I mention Susie, and that she sends her love.

"Who?"

"Susie. My friend who lives in San Francisco." I point to Susie's picture on Mary's wall, where many pictures of me and of Susie and Annie are pushed-pinned into it, so Mom can see familiar faces as she lies in bed.

"Oh, you mean the woman who looks like a movie star."

I laugh.

"Yea, Mom, the woman who looks like a movie star."

Susie's going to love hearing that.

DIRTY SEX

TUCSON, ARIZONA • WINTER, 2010

"You really don't have much experience with Sex, do you?"

I laugh.

"No, Mom, I have a quite a bit of experience with Sex."

"But mostly" she continues, "Just talking about it, not actually doing it, right?"

Smiling and laughing, I say, "No, No. Both talking and doing. A lot of both."

"Oh," she says, a bit puzzled and frustrated perhaps, that she is wrong about this.

"But you haven't had much Sex lately," Mary asks.

True.

"Yes, Mom, it's has been a while."

She looks very satisfied now, like she got me with that one, like she pinned me to the wall with my own recent bout of sexual abstinence.

"Well, you know your father and I..."

"Look over there! It's that nice picture of Susie!" I say, distracting her.

"She is such a pretty girl."

And that stopped that. I may be a very open minded man, but I'm not so open as to hear the details of my parents' sex life. Heard more than I wanted to know from Mom, two years ago while driving through New Mexico. Been there, done that, bought the T-shirt. But she's not quite done yet.

"Do you know what your father and I called it."

"No," I tentatively say, "I don't."

"We called it Dirty Sex."

She smiles.

MARY TALKING WITH VICTORIA

TUCSON, ARIZONA • SPRING, 2010

Mom's become sweet again, kind again. Even though it might not last, I like it. Like it a lot. Just last week she said she was sorry for something, and she really meant it. Really. Nice. It's tragic Mary had to get sick in order to become the mother I always wanted her to be. Good days and bad, we make each other laugh. (We Jenks can turn a phrase you know.) When she dies, I will truly miss her. I surely will.

We disconnected Mary's phone months ago. It's easier for friends to simply call the house phone, have the nurse on duty walk the phone over to Mom and have a conversation that way. Mom, who Dad used to joke, 'would be buried with her phone so she could call us from the other side,' can no longer figure out how to answer a telephone.

Some people call from North Carolina, but not many. My sister Pamela calls about once a week or so. But from the State of Virginia, where Mary was born and raised and lived the last 20 years of her life, none of her white friends, except two, call her at all. All of those people who stated loyalty and love for my parents have stopped calling. Granted, everyone liked Stuart more than Mary, and Mary tended to take people captive so she could put them to work, but that's no excuse, if you ask me. Don't tell me you love Mom, as she goes through this shit, and then just send her a Christmas card once a year, that she can't even read now.

I remember almost two years ago, right before we moved Mom to Tucson, we had a final dinner with Mary's white friends at a fish joint in Lively, Virginia. I was pissed just sitting there with crab and flounder on my plate. It took me a while to figure it out. The mood of her friends was 'Good riddance, Mary.'

I didn't get along with my mother back then either, but to have her supposedly good friends think that is truly fucked up. I don't care how much of a pain-in-the-neck Mom was. That's fucked up.

But there is one family and primarily one woman, the matriarch of that family, who have been loyal, helpful and kind to Mary and Stuart for years. That's Victoria. And her daughter Karen and her son Bunny, and frankly, all of her clan.

Victoria cleaned The River House for my parents for years. Came once a week to sweep the floor of my folks' place, on top of raising her own kids and grandkids, and working full time at Kentucky Fried Chicken. The River House really didn't need cleaning that much. It was just an excuse for my parents to give her money. Plus my Dad really loved her.

"We would sit on the front porch, and Stuart would tell me stories and we would laugh and laugh. Indeed we did." Victoria said.

And after Stuart died in 2001, she didn't go away. Even though she had her own health problems, either she or Karen would come weekly to clean the house. Mom moved to a smaller house in Mollusk, Virginia, and Karen still came and cleaned and washed the dishes.

Between 2003 and 2008, none of Mary's white friends called me to tell me that she was losing her mind. Nor did Victoria, but from her standing, it was out of her place to call. She was shocked, though, when I told her months ago, that no one communicated to me, my mother's odd new behaviors.

"Lordy, lordy. What is wrong with those people," she said.

"God damn White people. That's what's wrong." I said.

Victoria laughed. That wonderful loud laugh.

Victoria and her clan have lived in Nuttsville and thereabouts for generations. Her ancestors used to be slaves. They ain't no mo, but equality has yet to completely arrive in The Northern Neck of Virginia. Everyone else (everyone who is White) in the surrounding area has their mail delivered directly to their homes. Folks in Nuttsville have all their mail sent to a tiny post office and they have to go and pick it up.

Victoria, when she was a young girl, went to work for a rich White woman upriver a ways. 1950-something. She lasted until noon and then told that mean old White woman that 'I ain't going work for someone as spiteful as you.'

Boy, did I laugh when I first heard her tell that story.

She's a beautiful woman. Short and round with chocolate skin and a laugh that can rock the house. She, like my father, does not suffer fools well. Nor do I. I love her to death.

She and a number of her family have 'The Sugar.' Diabetes. Bunny had it bad, but is healing up. Victoria has been struggling with it for years, but now she has a long-standing gut pain coming from her pancreas that no one can figure out how to fix. She isn't going to die soon (fingers crossed) but she isn't living very happy either. She rarely complains and her children and grandchildren take good care of her. She lives in a small single-wide trailer, right on Route 354. It's good form to tap your horn as you drive by, unless it's late at night. I've honked dozens of times.

I love Victoria and she loves me. And she's loved my mother through thick and thin. And it isn't like she doesn't know Mary is an acquired taste. She knows. She also knows what Love is.

Last Christmas, I gave her a couple hundred dollars. It was nothing to Mom. It meant the world to Victoria. It made me happy to write the check.

Out of the blue, I sent a hundred more last month. Just so happened her well pump had recently broken and the money just about covered the cost.

"Praise the lord. Thank you, Stu," she said.

"Now, Victoria, I want you to know that Mary and I have a little bit of money and if you need a few hundred dollars at any time, I can easily write you a check," I said.

"Why, thank you, Stu. But I'm OK right now," she said.

"Well, just know it's there," I said.

"I sure appreciate it."

Bottom Line? She calls my mother at least once a week. Often times, Mom is sleeping or the nurse doesn't pick up because she's busy with another client. But she always calls. Always. Long distance from a land line.

Now, I've taken to carrying my cellphone in with me when I visit Mary and sometimes I call Victoria so she can talk with Mom while I'm there.

I had just told Mom I sent Victoria some money, and Mom was so excited to hear that we helped. I was too.

"Want to talk with her now? I can call her right now." I say.

"That would be wonderful," Mom says.

I dial the phone.

"Hello," I hear a husky voice on the other end. Tired, worn out.

"Hey, Victoria," I say.

"Hey!" she says loudly, brightening right up.

"How are you?" I say.

"I'm OK," she says, lying a little.

"I'm here with Mary. Would you like to talk with her?"

"I surely would." Victoria says.

I place the phone to Mom's ear, both of us holding the cell. I've turned up the volume on the earpiece. I can hear both sides of the conversation.

"Hello," Mom says.

"It's Victoria."

"Oh, I can't tell you how good it is to hear your voice," says Mary.

"It's so good to talk with you too. How are you, Ms. Jenks?"

"Well, today is a good morning. But...I'm sick, you know."

"I know," says Victoria.

"It's so good to hear your voice," Mom repeats.

"Thank you. And thank you for the very lovely Christmas gift," says Victoria.

"You're welcome. I hear Stu has sent you...some...more...money."

"Yes," she laughs as she says it, "It's very kind of him."

"Well, Victoria, I want you to know, if you ever need any money for anything, you just give me a call. OK?" says my mother.

"OK," I hear Victoria say. I can also hear that she's crying.

"That's so sweet of you, Ms. Jenks."

I'm misting up now too. Mom's not crying. She's here but not here, but her core generosity still lives on.

"Well, you know I love you, Victoria. I'm doing...well...I guess...OK... I guess."

Mom's losing the string of the conversation. She can't follow along for more than a minute or so now, whether in person or on the phone.

"I'm going to...go...now," says Mary. "Do you want to...talk with... Stu?"

"I sure do."

"I love you, Victoria."

"I love you too, Ms. Jenks."

"Here's Stu."

Mom lets go of the phone.

"Victoria, I'll call you later."

I can hear that Victoria is overwhelmed with joy. She can barely speak through the tears. I'm having a tough time too.

"OK, Stu," she says.

"And that check should get to you real soon."

"Thank you, Stu. Thank you."

"You're welcome, honey. And I'm always here if you need anything. I mean that," I say.

"I know you do."

"OK. I'll call you after I leave Momma."

"All right. Talk with you soon," she says.

"Love you."

"I love you too," says Victoria.

WHAT IS PRAYER?

GRACE CATHEDRAL, SAN FRANCISCO, CALIFORNIA
HOLY WEEK, 2010

"Help me out here, God," I say just before I type this sentence.

What am I really asking for? Well, I'm praying to be honest but not mean, transparent but not narcissistic, insightful but not arrogant, and most of all, not dull and boring in my writing.

But what is prayer? Who am I really praying to, and what do I really expect to receive?

First, What is God?

Succinctly, God is the Big Constant Energy of Good.

What isn't God to me?

God is not a huge consciousness that is specifically interested in Mr. Stu. God is not a gum ball machine that gives me candy when I've been good. God is not a Sleepy Old Man In The Sky who awakens from his slumber when he hears my prayers and then comes down and immediately does something about it. God is not a Bitter Old Man In A Cave who strikes down those who have wronged me. God isn't even a kind benevolent force who in its infinite Love, protects me from all harm and heals those I love, just because it can. No. God is not that to me either.

God is just Goodness. Always there. A 60-cycle hum of Love. An electrical socket of Light and Healing. A living, growing energy in all things: plants, animals, minerals, the Sky, the Moon and the Stars. And God is in me and in you, too. Goodness lives inside of us, outside of us, not in our totality, but a growing part of all of us: The quiet still voice that guides him throughout his day, not the loud ego that needs to be right. The loving glance at a stranger as she sees the God in them, not the judgmental glare at a driver who just cut her off. The warm touch of a lover's hand in his, not the harsh yank to a three-year-old's arm.

God is Love. God is Light. God is Healing. God is Good.

So when I pray to God, what do I expect? Not much. What do I hope for? A lot. An awful lot. Seem contradictory? It's not. A teacher taught me 25 years ago, that any two contradictory truths make a paradox, and hence create an even larger absolute. Do I pray for miracles? Not often. Do I wish for miracles to happen? You bet I do. But do I pray for God to intercede? No. I don't believe in an Interventionist God. But do I pray for Grace in my life. Yes, I do.

Christina Grof once said, "You will never be abused by a spiritual experience." I don't believe I'm a chess piece on God's board.

So what do I mean when I say, 'You are in my prayers' like I say quite often to family members who are sick, or to friends who are scared, and to people who are hurt?

I mean simply this: That I love you and that I'm thinking about you, hoping for the very best, and if the worst comes, I'll be there. In spades.

I'm not praying for the Sleepy Old Man to look down from his cloud and wave a wand and your cancer goes away. I'm not praying to the Gum Ball Machine to give you some cash. I'm not praying to a Big Personal Thing to listen only to me.

I'm simply saying: I love you, and I'm here and I believe God's here too.

That's it. But that's a lot, isn't it?

I believe it was Jean Houston who said, "Through human beings' good acts, God grows."

I'm watering God as he waters me. Or something like that.

And when I pray to God, to help me be a better man, to help me stay sober another day, to help me quit smoking someday, to help me be there for my mother as she dies, to help me be loving to those who don't like me, to help me be loving to those who really like me a lot, to help me be present, right here, right now, in all I do and see and know; I'm not asking God to fix it, or to intervene, or to make it all better through his will alone. I'm praying that the Little God in me connects with the Big God out there, and that as we commune through my daily practices of prayer, meditation, good deeds and the washing of dishes, I become a healthier man, a more giving and tolerant man, and a better human being on the planet.

My friend Craig puts it best. It comes down to two small words.

"Be nice," he says.

MARY ON THE FOURTH OF JULY

TUCSON, ARIZONA • SUMMER, 2010

"Now that's just stupid," Mary says.

She's unhappy that I won't have sex with her. She's had this desire, off and on, for the past few months. I tell her again that I'm her son and she's my mother, but that doesn't change her mind. I bring up Dad, who she had a healthy sex life with, to distract her from her randy line of thinking, but it doesn't work this time. She's angrily asked, in the past, 'What books is that written in?" when she's wanted to have sex with me, and I've refused, and I've politely said, 'It's in a lot of books, Mom. The Bible. The Koran. The Tao, I guess. All the Native American oral traditions. Pretty much in all the books.' Mary just hurumps when I turn her down. Mom never had good boundaries, to begin with and now, with half her brain gone from dementia, she has none. Like a little girl who wants what she wants when she wants it.

"Mom, I'm not going to do that," I says. "Now, when you get close to death, I'll be by your bed side a lot, but I won't be sleeping with you."

I touch her hand. It's not what she wants. Ain't going to happen, Mom.

I push her in her wheelchair from her bedroom back to the head of the dining room table where I found her when I arrived today. She loves sitting at the head of the table at Crossroads, a high-end adult care home where she's lived for going on two years now, with the nine other residents who range from those who can't speak from their advanced Alzheimer's to others who are just too depressed to respond. And then there's Mary: chatty, demanding, outgoing, polite sometimes, openly judgmental other times. The staff at Crossroads loves her because she actually talks and is kind of funny, but much of Mary's dialogue lost its humor for me years ago. But I do feel sad that she suffers so. Anxious, confused, in a world that's only as big as the room she's currently in. I do pray for her eminent death, but only God knows when that's going to happen, and I think He's puzzled about when Mary's going to die.

I give Mary a kiss on her forehead and tell her I'll call her from the road every day. I remind her I'll be gone for a week or so. She doesn't hear this, but tries another tact instead.

"I just want to have you to touch in the middle of the night is all," she says.

Yeah, Mom. I tried that tactic too with women in the past. They didn't believe me then. I don't believe you now.

"I love you, Mom," I say. "I'll call you tomorrow."

I give her another kiss on her forehead and exit out the front door.

I'M HERE

TUCSON, ARIZONA • SUMMER, 2010

"They shouldn't even let you in the door," Mary said last month, when she first saw my bleach blond hair

"Stu, she's crazy!" Mary says every time I speak her daughter Pamela's name.

"If that's the best you can do, you shouldn't even try," Mary said a while back, shaming me like she has done for years, but now a bit playfully. I don't take it on.

"When are you going to undress?" Mary asked yesterday, still trying to get her hands in my pants.

"Not for a good long while," I said, "Not until I get home." Mom looked disappointed.

Been trying to get 'The Transpersonal Papers' to the printer these last couple months. A week away from delivering it to Gail, my book designer. That's my excuse for not writing about Mary lately.

But closer to the truth is that Mary's painfully slow decline toward Death isn't quite as cute and funny as it was a year ago. Now, it's just tragic. For her. Me? It's just hard to watch and harder to write about.

But I'm here. And I'll continue to be here. That's what I do. The same thing billions of sons have done over the last 50,000 years for a dying parent.

I'm here, to be with you, as you die.

WELL, LET'S NOT GO THAT FAR

TUCSON, ARIZONA • SUMMER, 2010

I woke Mary up. It's around 7:30 on a Saturday night. Joseph, the night nurse, just left after giving Mom her meds. She flirted with him a bit. He's a tall, young, handsome Nigerian man. If I were gay, I'd flirt with him too.

Mom is in the best mood. She's smiling and laughing and she's making me laugh too. She's following the conversation or at least pretending to. What a delight. I never know what I'm walking into, when I visit Mom, and this is a welcome surprise.

"So Mom, I'm thinking about dedicating the new book to you. Well, maybe," I say, pulling her leg just a little.

She smiles and says, "Well wouldn't that be nice?" and then laughs. And I laugh too.

"Mom, you still want to die, right?"

"Oh no, I want to live," she says, with only half-hearted earnestness.

"Really? You wanted to die yesterday," I say.

She looks a little puzzled.

"I just don't like that you suffer so," I say.

"Well, I do suffer," she says matter-of-factly.

"But it's OK if you want to live..." I continue.

(Truly, I hope she dies soon. Watching her suffer hurts. Quite a lot.)

"...it's OK," I say. "We have enough money for at least two more years."

She smiles as big as I've seen her smile in a year. She looks right straight at me and says:

"Well, let's not go that far."

She laughs. She knows she's told a great joke. I laugh too. Then she laughs again, and then I laugh and laugh and laugh some more. And so does she.

THE BIG NOT-FUN

TUCSON, ARIZONA • SUMMER, 2010

There's a screamer in the house now. The nurse says they'll be soon moving her to the locked dementia house across the courtyard, but my guess is they'll have to wait for someone to die first, over there.

'It's so good to see you' upon my arrival, has been replaced with 'Where have you been?' 'I love you, Stu" as I leave, with 'Why are you going?' Mom has a new look in her eye: everything confuses her, even the sight of me. Her attention is quickly pulled to every sound in the house, from the loud shouts of the screamer to the dull drones of commercials on the living room TV. Even when I'm alone with her in her bedroom, she barely tracks what I'm saying most days. A car outside can break her attention, and she's gone.

It's right before dinner. Mary's spilled her drink. I get up to find a paper towel. The nurse shows me the rag pile. I grab one and whip up the spilled apple juice. I tell Mom that I just went to the post office to mail one of my books, and now I'm on my way to the studio and I thought I'd drop by to see her, since she's on the way.

"We're going to the post office," she yells to the nurse, who's making dinner in the kitchen.

"No, Mom. I just went to the post office."

"Stu and the post office," she shouts.

"Mom. It's OK. The nurse is busy."

She turns her head and looks me square in the face. I see very little behind her eyes. Confusion, a little fear, very little recognition, of me or anything else.

I sigh.

We're firmly in The Big Not-Fun now, aren't we, Mom?

MARY'S PLASTIC LEI

TUCSON, ARIZONA • SUMMER, 2010

Mary and I talk for a while. Actually, I talk and she barely says anything at all, but when Mary does speak, it's filled with sweetness and love for me. She is having a good day. No, that's not it. She's having good moments while I'm here today. The rest of her day and tonight, after I'm gone, will consist of her sleeping a lot, feeling perpetually scared, eating a couple small meals, perhaps vacantly gazing at the TV at some point, and then talking gibberish to herself while she lies in bed. Truly, I am the only bright spot in her day. Not because I'm wonderful or special or anything, but simply because I'm her son, and I have come to visit.

As I drive home to my apartment, I think about our pets. If I had a dog or a cat, who couldn't walk anymore, who barely ate anything, who seemed to recognize me sometimes but not at other times, who was very frightened and confused all the time, and who was a very old dog or cat, what would I do? I would tell her I loved her, and I would take her to the vet and have her put to sleep. But what do we do to our demented and terminally-sick elderly in America? We give them drugs and feed them food that keeps them alive. We hire people to change their diapers, to spoon-feed them and to then put them to bed or wheel them in front of a television screen. And we wait for them to die. But due, in my mind, to a perverted misinterpretation of Judeo-Christian ethics, we can't give them a large dose of morphine until they are in immense pain or filled with cancer. We just keep feeding them, cleaning them, drugging them until Death comes.

And I know if I stop visiting my mother all together and leave her all alone in her own private hell, she would most likely die sooner rather than later. But I can't do that, even though I know it would hasten her end. It would just be too cruel. But I have thought about it.

Nor can I sneak into her room, late at night, with a syringe full of opiates and inject her while she sleeps, then sending her to see her husband or whoever or whatever is on the other side. But sometimes, sometimes, I sure wish somebody would give her that injection.

A late-afternoon rainbow shines over the Catalina Mountains. I weakly smile.

I'll see Mary tomorrow or the next day. I am, after all, the only joy she has.

FLAME SPIRAL FOR THE HOPI CLOWNS

WUPATKI, ARIZONA • SUMMER, 2010

Was up on First Mesa at lunchtime. Watched thirty Hopi women in beautiful fringed shawls carry pallets of pies and boxes of pika bread to the Kachina Dancers, who were on break. Went down the hill later to speak with Connie and her husband in Polacca. He had a heart attack three weeks ago. One stent's already in. One or two more to go.

"It's in the hands of the big guy upstairs now," he said. He looked scared. I'm frightened for him too.

I've found my spot now, leaning against an alley wall, peaking around the corner into the village square. I can see everything.

A Mudhead bangs a slow rhythm on his drum. Fifty Kachina Dancers chant and dance, shifting their weight from side to side. The Kachinas' chants sound more like what Tibetan monks sing, than something you'd hear at a Pow-wow. The women of Middle Village sit on folding chairs, listening and laughing. Six Hopi Clowns spit from a roof top, onto one person in particular in the square. The Clowns then repel down a rope and continue their playful abuse. The drum, the chants, the dancing, the laughter, create a hole in this World, and the Breath of Gods from the Outside, fills the mesa.

I laugh at the Clowns' jokes. I cry with the joy of The Holy Breeze. And then I laugh and cry, all at the same time.

THE VIEW OUT MARY'S WINDOW

TUCSON, ARIZONA • FALL, 2010

Often, in the past, Mary would lose her train of thought when a car would pass outside her window. She'd follow the car with her eyes and then her eyes would return to center. She'd then stare into the distance, at nothing, at everything, or at something only she could see.

She doesn't look out her window much anymore. Now, you might find her sitting in her wheelchair at the dining room table, watching the staff cook in the kitchen. Or she might be reclined in the La-Z-Boy in the living room, blankly viewing the flat screen on the wall. Or she might be in bed, quietly chatting with people I can't see: her mother, her husband, her high school and church friends. I occasional catch snippets of her conversations as I approach her room. Her voice, weak and mumbled, happy and pitiful, all at the same time. She stops talking altogether when I enter her room.

A Dodge van rolls by. I don't follow it with my eyes. I just gaze at the red Bougainvillea outside Mom's window and then stare down that street that leads to the east.

WHY?

TUCSON, ARIZONA • THANKSGIVING, 2010

"What...I...can't...understand," says Mary, "is why?"

"Why?....Why?....Why?....Why?"

She's stuck on a word. This happens a lot now. Her breathing's very shallow too. She's not particularly anxious today but she appears weak. Other family members talk to their demented loved ones on the other side of the living room. One of the caregivers waits in the kitchen for everyone to leave before serving the turkey. This is wise.

Meals at Crossroads Adult Care Center are not a pretty sight, with seven invalids struggling to find their mouths with their forks.

"Well, Mom, Why is not my favorite word. I've found that it's pretty futile trying to figure out Why, and if I do find the answer to Why, it doesn't really seem to help that much."

Mom looks at my face as if it's the Moon, with a look of awe that isn't really warranted, but I'm happy that the sight of me brings her pleasure. The easiest loving thing I do, visiting Mary.

"Yeah, so don't worry about the Why, Mom. But the What and Where is I'll see you tomorrow."

She smiles.

"You...have...such...beautiful...teeth," Mary says.

THE BIG ORANGE CHRISTMAS BALL

SOLSTICE ROCK, ARIZONA • WINTER SOLSTICE, 2010

Today's a good day, but yesterday, Mary was terrified. Wide-eyed, a little cruel, a lot scared. Last thing she yelled to me as I walked out the door was 'You're abandoning me!'

"Mary, do you know who I am?" I say today, as I sit down on her bed.

"You know...I...do...not."

"I'm your son."

"I won't...have known that," she says.

"That's OK, Mom. I know who you are."

I repeat to Mary her personal current events, like I do most visits. You've be deathly ill for over two years. We thought you were dying a year ago, but you didn't. I live ten miles away. I won't die before you. Everything is taken care of. You'll be buried in Virginia. You don't have to stay alive on my account. It's been hard for me to watch you suffer. These hard facts always seem to calm Mary down, giving her a momentary connection to her past life of church, telephone calls, family and friends within this current life of eat, sleep, pee and poop. And always now, an opaque cloud of wakeful dreaming hangs in the air, an indoor storm that hardly makes sense to her or to me. She speaks a little. I say a lot. She's very happy to see me, but I'm still not sure she knows I'm her son.

After fifteen minutes of this and that, I prepare to leave. I stand up.

"Your father was here...last night," Mary says.

I guess she does know it's me.

"No kidding," I say. "Did he stay with you?"

"He came in...and did his thing."

She smiles. I don't ask what his thing is, but I'm pretty sure I know.

"And he stayed...with me."

"He spent the night with you?" I ask.

Mom nods.

"I'm so happy, Mom. I've been asking Dad to come over and lend a hand. That's great."

"I've been seeing him...a lot...lately," Mary says.

"Ah," I sigh. "That's so great."

Mary may be getting closer to going over.

"You know I feel Dad too, sometimes." I say. "I talk with him from time to time. You can ask him to come over and sleep with you anytime you like."

She looks puzzled with the asking part.

"Or he'll just come on his own. I really hope he comes and sleeps with you tonight," I say.

"Me...too," says Mary.

I kiss Mom's forehead. She weakly kisses my cheek. I leave her room.

> 'At times I see you/ You silver rider/
> Sometimes your voice is not enough.
> Your face in windows/ Outside forever/
> Nobody dreamed you'd save the world.'
> "Silver Rider" by Alan Sparhawk
> and Mimi Parker of Low

Been coming up here to pray on the Solstice for over 20 years. Drawn flame spirals up here, prayed for light, cried for the suffering, even felt a little sorry for myself a few times, but always I've felt better on the drive down the hill. You can see the Rock from the road if you know where to look, but most don't, they're more focused on getting to the top of Mt. Lemmon. It's a special rock to me, but not to many others. That's fine. Everybody's got their Rock. This is one of mine.

A few times, I've had to pray lower on the mountain or on another hill, due to snow and ice on the road, but tonight, no snow's on the ground and mostly clear skies above me, with a lunar eclipse in North America's and my future.

Tripod in the truck. 70-200mm with the 2x extender rests on the front passenger seat. I'm late.

Every other Solstice, I'm here by myself. Not tonight. Parked cars sit in almost every turnout as I ascend The Catalina Highway. The full eclipse is coming fast. Most of the Moon is gone. Yikes.

I sing along to a Low song as I drive. Buddy Miller plays the lead. Robert Plants sings it. It's a perfect night.

I find my turnout. Park. Grab. Go.

Five minutes later, I'm setting up the tripod, attaching the 5D Mark II, plugging in the cable release, composing the shot. Looks like I have a few minutes before totality. I start my Solstice prayers but stop them, delightfully distracted by the magic overhead. It'll wait.

Then the white Full Moon is gone, replaced by an orange globe. I bet I'm not the only North American who thinks it looks like a Christmas ball.

I lie down on the granite rock, gazing up at a great sea of stars where only a hour ago, hardly any stars were visible in the Full Moon light. The cable release rest in my right hand. I click away dozens of exposures. My gut tells me I have the one I need in the can.

I stand and begin to pray. At Solstice Rock, I pray aloud.

"Well, God, you know how I do this. I come up here every year and pray for everybody. Tonight, I'm a little self conscious for I know this year's praying will be the last story in the Dementia book. I'll try and not be all spiritual and shit." I chuckle. "Well, screw that."

I look up at the shrouded Moon. Like an orange transparent curtain in front of a bright light.

"Maybe I'll pray for everyone to have the curtain pulled away. Nah. I just want Mary to go to the other side. That's why I'm thinking this curtain shit. It's really not up to me when Mom dies, is it, God? She's on her own little journey now. I've been there for part of it, but it's her thing. No. Something else I need to pray for."

I crane my neck to see the Moon. I realize it's much easier to look at it if I'm lying down. Never solstice-prayed on my back before. First time for everything.

I settle in, lying on my back again. Such a wondrous and singular sight. The sky full of stars, like on a New Moon night, but there is that Christmas ball glowing directly overhead. I am so lucky. I am so thankful. Thankful.

"God, this year I want to give thanks to all my friends, all my acquaintances, all my co-workers. And all of those In The Rooms."

I name them all, one by one, as best I can.

"And I don't mean I simply express gratitude for their love and care. I mean to give them the gift of thanks. That they may feel thankful for what they have, both good and bad. Yeah. Thankful for the bad. Now, that's the hard one, isn't it. I don't do that, that well. Nobody does. And I don't want to do some spiritual bypass, some woo woo trick fuck, that minimizes the pain that sometimes comes from being a human. No. I mean something like, even as we go through trials and sufferings and losses and griefs, that we don't get swallowed up in the crap and lose sight of the wonders and joys around us. To remember that we're alive, that there is always hope for happiness. That if I'm sick, that I still have good overall health, and people who love me, and a warm place to sleep tonight. That when love is gone, it was there before it left and it will return; It'll just look and feel like someone else. To know that we Americans tend to be the financially wealthiest people on the planet yet we take those riches for granted. I know I do sometimes."

"God, I'm so lucky. So grateful. So thankful. I've been able to live the dream this past year of being a full time artist, and I gotta tell you, doing this full time makes the job a lot easier. I'll do this until the money runs out, or maybe it won't run out. Either way, I am living a wonderful life. I can't tell you how happy I am, God."

I stand up. I look toward the city lights of Tucson, below me to the South.

"So, God, give thanks those I know and love. To all in Tucson. To all in Arizona. To all in the West. To all Americans. To everyone in the World."

"And thank you, God. Thank you."

I look toward the zenith again. Still the big orange Moon. Still the big orange Christmas ball.

Still.

ACKNOWLEDGEMENTS

Many thanks to Team Fezziwig: Gail Cross, Annie Gordon, Ken Backer, Bo Petersen, Cathy Spann, Nathan Bardsley, Charles de Lint, Craig Acorn, Michael Doll and Dirk Matthews.

And continued thanks to all of the staff and owners at Crossroads Adult Care Center, who take such good care of my mother; to Casa de la Luz Hospice for preparing my mother for death; to Tri-Care For Life & Medicare for paying for some of Mary's care; and to Ed Pittman of the Bank of Lancaster for managing Mary's money so well these last ten years.

And lastly, I thank the mysterious spirits that guide me to do the right thing. Part the God within, part the God without, part something totally inexplicable. Without this Holy Ghost, I would be lost.

PHOTOGRAPHY CREDITS:

All images are by Stu Jenks.

(To purchase prints or image rights of any of these photographs, contact Stu via email at stujenks@gmail.com. All rights reserved.)

Cover:	"Mary On The Fourth Of July" © 2010
Page 41:	"The Pine Forest Spiral" © 2001
Page 42:	"The Javelina Skull Spiral" © 2001
	"Stu And Stuart Sleeping" © 2001
Page 43:	"Harriman, Tennessee" © 2008
Page 44:	"Mary At The Cadillac Ranch" © 2008
	"After The Arkansas Incident" © 2008
Page 45:	"Bristlecone Hoop Dance" © 2009
	"Bristlecone Before The Dance" © 2009
Page 46:	"Mary Talking With Victoria" © 2010
	"Shoot You Myself" © 2009
	"Dirty Sex" © 2010
Page 47:	"Tearful Mary" © 2009
	"Mary Sees" © 2009
Page 48:	"I Want My Momma" © 2009
	"Mr. Let-Us-Pray" © 2010
	"Mary 4.0" © 2009
Page 49:	"At The End Of The Hall" © 2010
Page 50:	"Mary's Anxious Hands" © 2010
Page 51:	"Mary And Pamela" © 2007
	"Mary, Pamela And Virginia" © 2009
Page 52:	"Milkshake Mary" © 2010
Page 53:	"Courtney Saum" © 2009
	"Mary Sees, Again" © 2009
Page 54:	"Solstice Rock, Arizona" © 1998
	"Sage Grouse Flame Spirals" © 2010
Page 55:	"Mary At Christmastime" © 2010
Page 56:	"Give Thanks Lunar Eclipse" © 2010